STROKE

A Doctor's Practical Guide to Prevention & Early Detection

Dr Prabhat Das

MD, PhD, FACP

Better Health with Dr Das Series

Hardcover ISBN: 978-1-971672-61-8

Paperback ISBN: 978-1-971672-60-1

eBook ISBN: 978-1-971672-59-5

Printed in the United States of America

Disclaimer

This book is intended solely for educational and informational purposes. It is not meant to replace personal medical advice, diagnosis, or treatment.

Although I am a licensed physician, reading this book does not establish a doctor-patient relationship. Each individual's health condition, medical history, and risk factors are unique. Any medical decision should be made in partnership with your own healthcare professional who understands your specific situation.

Medical science is continually advancing. New research and updated guidelines may lead to changes in recommendations over time.

TABLE OF CONTENTS:

About the Author

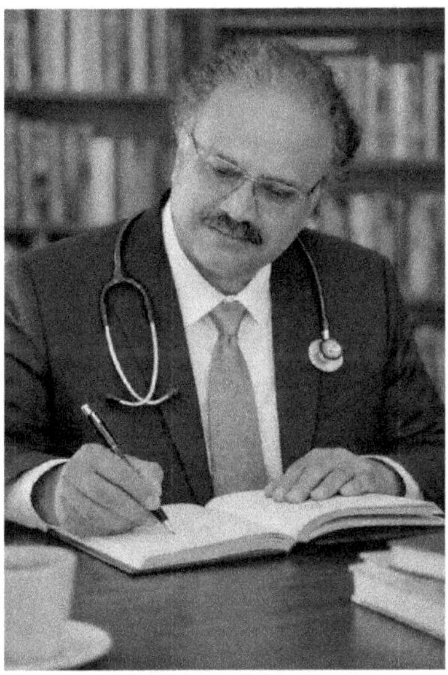

I am Dr Prabhat Das, MD, PhD, FACP. My journey in medicine began in India and, over the past thirty-five years, has continued in the United States, where I have had the privilege of caring for patients across a wide range of medical settings. I am trained in Internal Medicine, Pulmonary Diseases, and Critical Care. For me, medicine has never been just a profession. It has been a lifelong commitment shaped by learning, service, and a deep respect for the trust patients place in their physician.

Over the years, I have had the honor of caring for patients in many different situations. I have seen individuals in my office for routine concerns, treated urgent conditions in busy emergency rooms, managed serious illnesses in the hospital, and cared for critically ill patients in intensive care units. Each setting has taught me something valuable. Each patient has added to my understanding of what it truly means to care for another human being.

But one lesson has stood above all others. Medicine is not only about tests, diagnoses, or treatments. It is about people. It is about listening carefully, understanding fears that are often left unspoken, and guiding patients through uncertainty with clarity and compassion. Again and again, I have seen that what people want most is simple, trustworthy information. They want to understand what is happening in their bodies. They want to feel confident about the decisions they are making for their health and for their families.

These experiences have deeply shaped how I think about health, illness, prevention, and the human side of healing.

That is the reason behind the '**Better Health with Dr Das Series'**. Through these books, I hope to reach individuals I may never meet in person but who are searching for clear and reliable guidance. In today's world, health information is everywhere, yet much of it is confusing, overwhelming, and sometimes misleading. My goal is to cut through that noise and present important medical topics in a way that is simple, practical, and reassuring.

Every page of this series is guided by two foundations: reliable scientific knowledge and decades of real-world clinical experience. I want you, the reader, to feel informed, confident, and empowered. Not overwhelmed. Not confused. But clear about what you can do, step by step, to improve your health.

If even one reader feels less anxious, more informed, or better prepared to take control of their health after reading these books, then this work has served its purpose.

Helping people live healthier, longer, more confident and better-informed lives remains one of the greatest privileges of my life.

CHAPTER 1: Stroke: The Brain Attack You Cannot Afford to Ignore

Why This Chapter Matters

A stroke does not announce itself politely. It arrives suddenly, often in the middle of an ordinary moment.

I have seen patients who were talking normally one minute and struggling to speak the next. I have seen families sitting together at dinner when one person suddenly cannot lift a hand or smile properly.

In those moments, knowledge becomes life-saving.

This chapter is not just an introduction. It is the foundation of everything that follows. If you understand this chapter well, you will never look at stroke casually again.

What Is a Stroke

A stroke occurs when blood flow to a part of the brain is suddenly interrupted.

The brain depends on a constant supply of oxygen and nutrients. Blood carries these through a network of arteries. When this supply stops, even briefly, brain cells begin to suffer.

There are two main ways this happens.

A blood vessel may become blocked, stopping blood flow to the brain.

Or a blood vessel may rupture, causing bleeding inside the brain.

In both situations, the result is the same. Brain cells are injured, and if treatment is delayed, some of them die.

This is why stroke is a true emergency.

Stroke Is a Brain Attack

Most people understand the seriousness of a heart attack. When blood flow to the heart is blocked, the heart muscle is damaged.

Stroke is very simiar, but the organ involved is the brain.

That is why stroke is often called a brain attack.

The brain controls movement, speech, memory, vision, balance, swallowing, emotions, and judgment. When stroke damages any part of the brain, the effects can be immediate and life-changing.

This is not a condition to watch and wait.

This is a condition to act on.

Doctor's Pearl

Think of stroke the same way you think of a heart attack. Immediate action saves function, and often saves life.

WHAT HAPPENS IN A STROKE

A stroke occurs when the blood supply to a part of the brain is interrupted or when a blood vessel breaks.

NORMAL BLOOD FLOW

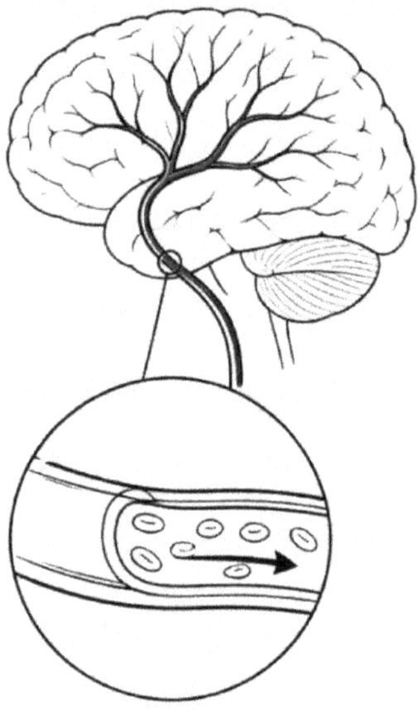

Blood flows freely to the brain.

STROKE (INTERRUPTED FLOW)

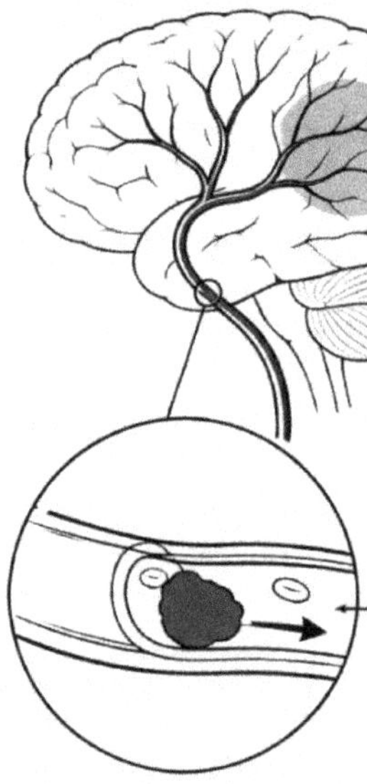

Blood clot blocks the artery.

Blood flow is blocked. Brain cells do not get oxygen and begin to die.

BLOCKED ARTERY
(Ischemic Stroke)

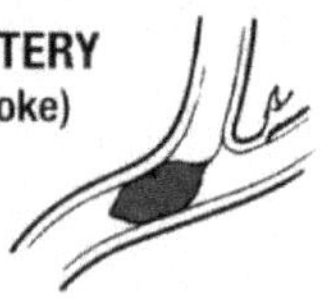

BLEEDING VESSEL
(Hemorrhagic Stroke)

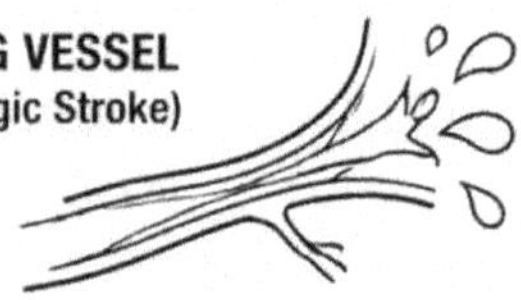

Quick action can save brain cells.
Time lost is brain lost.

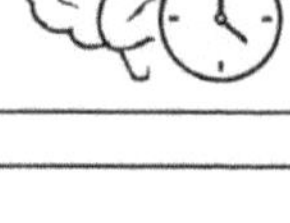

Time Is Brain

There is one concept I want you to remember throughout this book.

Time is brain.

When blood flow stops, brain cells begin to lose oxygen. Some cells die within minutes. Others are at risk but can still be saved if treatment is given quickly.

This creates a narrow window of opportunity.

If a patient reaches the hospital early, doctors may be able to restore blood flow, limit damage, and improve recovery.

If there is delay, that opportunity may be lost.

This is why hesitation is dangerous.

Do not wait for symptoms to improve.
Do not try home remedies.
Do not delay.

Call 911.

Why Stroke Is So Important

Stroke is one of the leading causes of disability worldwide. It affects millions of people and changes lives in an instant.

But beyond numbers, stroke has a human impact.

It affects independence. It affects families. It affects the ability to walk, talk, think clearly, and live a normal life.

In my practice, I have seen patients who return to near-normal life after timely treatment. I have also seen patients who suffer severe disability because of delay.

The difference is often measured in minutes.

The Encouraging Truth: Stroke Can Often Be Prevented

Here is the most hopeful part.

Many strokes can be prevented.

Stroke is rarely a random event. It is often the result of long-standing risk factors such as high blood pressure, diabetes, high cholesterol, smoking, and unhealthy lifestyle.

These conditions quietly damage blood vessels over time.

But they can be controlled.

Blood pressure can be managed.
Diabetes can be controlled.
Cholesterol can be treated.
Smoking can be stopped.
Physical activity can be increased.

Small, steady changes can make a powerful difference.

Who Should Pay Special Attention

This book is especially important if you:

Have high blood pressure, diabetes, or high cholesterol

Have a history of smoking

Are overweight or physically inactive

Have atrial fibrillation or heart disease

Have a family history of stroke

Have already had a TIA or stroke

Even if none of these apply, awareness is still valuable. Stroke can occur in anyone.

Myth vs Fact

Myth: Stroke happens only to very old people
Fact: Risk increases with age, but stroke can occur at any age

Myth: Stroke always causes severe paralysis
Fact: Some strokes begin with mild or subtle symptoms that are often ignored

Myth: If symptoms improve, there is no problem
Fact: Temporary symptoms may be a warning sign of a more serious stroke ahead

Common Mistakes to Avoid

Waiting to see if symptoms improve

Ignoring mild or unusual symptoms

Trying home remedies instead of seeking help

Driving to the hospital instead of calling 911

Stopping medications without medical advice

These mistakes are common. They are also preventable.

A Real-Life Perspective

I remember a patient in his early sixties. He developed mild speech difficulty and slight weakness in his hand. He thought it was fatigue and decided to rest.

By the time he reached the hospital, several hours had passed. The opportunity for certain treatments was gone.

In contrast, another patient with similar symptoms called 911 immediately. He received early treatment and recovered with minimal disability.

The difference was not luck.

It was awareness and action.

Key Points

Stroke is a sudden interruption of blood flow to the brain

It can be caused by blockage or bleeding

Brain cells are damaged quickly when blood flow stops

Time is critical in treatment

Early action improves recovery

Many strokes can be prevented by controlling risk factors

Chapter Summary

Stroke is a medical emergency that affects the brain and can lead to serious disability or death if not treated quickly. It occurs when blood flow to the brain is interrupted, either by a blockage or by bleeding.

The most important concept is that time matters. Early recognition and immediate action can significantly improve outcomes. At the same time, many strokes can be prevented by managing risk factors such as blood pressure, diabetes, cholesterol, and lifestyle habits.

Understanding stroke is the first step toward protecting yourself and your family.

Action Plan

- Think of stroke as a brain attack that requires immediate action
- Decide now that you will call 911 if symptoms occur
- Begin monitoring your blood pressure if you have risk factors
- Discuss your personal stroke risk with your doctor
- Share this knowledge with your family
- Never ignore even mild or temporary symptoms

Bridge to Chapter 2

Now that you clearly understand what stroke is and why it is so urgent, the next step is to understand that not all strokes are the same.

In the next chapter, we will explore the different types of stroke and why this distinction matters for treatment and recovery.

CHAPTER 2: The Three Faces of Stroke: Clot, Bleeding, and the Warning Stroke

Why This Chapter Matters

In the previous chapter, we understood that stroke is a brain emergency.

Now we take the next important step.

Stroke is not one single condition. It has different forms, and each form behaves differently, is treated differently, and carries different risks.

This is not just academic knowledge. It explains why doctors act so quickly and why certain treatments are given in some patients but not in others.

For you, the most important point is simple.

You do not need to identify the type of stroke at home. You only need to recognize the symptoms and act immediately.

Still, understanding these types will help you appreciate how critical early care really is.

Ischemic Stroke: The Most Common Type

Most strokes are ischemic strokes.

This type occurs when a blood vessel supplying the brain becomes blocked.

Think of a pipe that becomes clogged. Blood cannot reach that part of the brain. Without oxygen, brain cells begin to suffer.

This blockage is usually caused by a blood clot.

There are two main ways these clots form.

First, the clot can form within the artery itself. Over time, high blood pressure, diabetes, and high cholesterol damage the inner lining of blood vessels. Fatty deposits build up, narrow the artery, and create a surface where clots can form.

Second, the clot can form elsewhere, often in the heart, and then travel to the brain. This is called an embolic stroke. A common cause is an irregular heart rhythm known as atrial fibrillation.

Doctor's Pearl

In ischemic stroke, the goal is urgent and clear. Restore blood flow as quickly as possible.

Hemorrhagic Stroke: When a Vessel Ruptures

The second type of stroke is hemorrhagic stroke.

Here, the problem is bleeding.

A blood vessel in the brain ruptures, and blood leaks into or around the brain tissue. This damages the brain and increases pressure inside the skull.

Although less common than ischemic stroke, hemorrhagic stroke is often more severe.

The most common cause is long-standing high blood pressure, which weakens blood vessels over time.

Other causes include aneurysms, abnormal blood vessels, and certain medications.

Some patients describe a sudden, severe headache, often unlike anything they have felt before.

Treatment is very different from ischemic stroke. Instead of dissolving a clot, the focus is on controlling the bleeding and protecting the brain.

Myth vs Fact

Myth: All strokes are caused by blocked arteries
Fact: Some strokes are caused by bleeding, and the treatment is completely different

Transient Ischemic Attack: The Warning Stroke

The third type is called a transient ischemic attack, or TIA.

Many people call it a mini-stroke, but this term can be misleading.

A TIA occurs when blood flow to the brain is temporarily interrupted. Symptoms appear suddenly, just like a stroke, but they resolve within minutes or hours.

Because the symptoms go away, many people ignore them.

This is a serious mistake.

A TIA is often a warning sign that a major stroke may occur soon. The risk is highest in the first few days after a TIA.

You should treat a TIA as an emergency.

Common Mistake to Avoid

Saying, "It went away, so it must be nothing."

A TIA is often the body's early warning signal. Ignoring it can lead to a more serious event.

Understanding the Differences in Simple Terms

Let us simplify the three types.

Ischemic stroke
Caused by a blocked artery

Hemorrhagic stroke
Caused by bleeding in the brain

TIA
A temporary interruption of blood flow and a warning sign

Even though the causes are different, the symptoms often look similar.

That is why you should never try to decide the type at home.

Your role is to act quickly.

THREE TYPES OF STROKE

Strokes happen in different ways.
Understanding the type helps in the right treatment.

1. ISCHEMIC STROKE
(Blocked Artery)

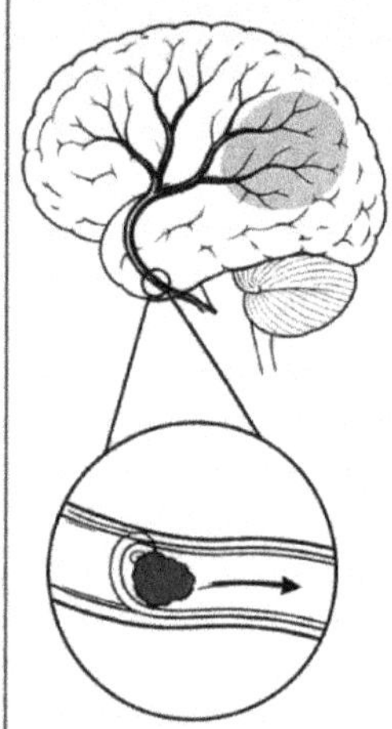

A blood clot blocks an artery in the brain. The brain cells do not get blood and oxygen.

Most common type

2. HEMORRHAGIC STROKE
(Bleeding in the Brain)

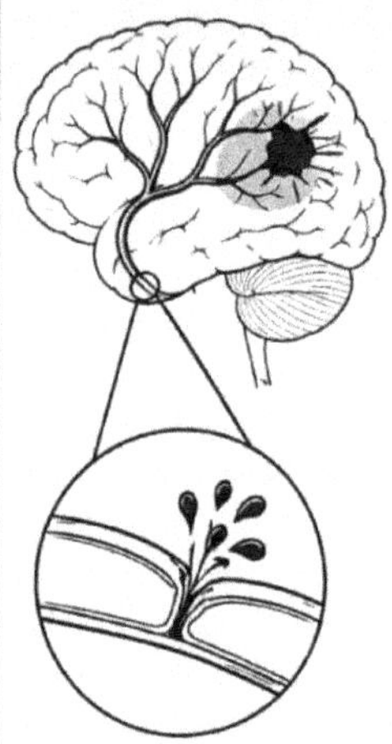

A blood vessel in the brain bursts and causes bleeding. This increases pressure and damages brain cells.

Can be life threatening

3. TIA
(Mini Stroke)

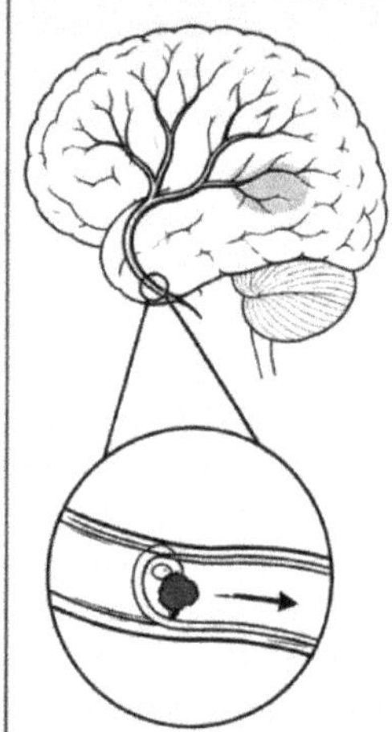

A temporary blockage stops blood flow for a short time. Symptoms disappear within minutes to hours.

Warning sign of future stroke

**Know the type. Act fast.
Protect the brain. Save life.**

Why This Matters in Real Life

When a patient reaches the hospital, doctors must quickly determine the type of stroke.

This decision guides treatment.

For example:

- Clot-dissolving treatment can help in ischemic stroke
- The same treatment can be dangerous in hemorrhagic stroke

This is why rapid imaging is done immediately.

Time is saved. Treatment is targeted.

A Real-Life Example

Two patients arrive with similar symptoms such as weakness and difficulty speaking.

One has a blocked artery. The other has bleeding in the brain.

Their symptoms look similar, but their treatments are completely different.

This is why early hospital care is essential.

Key Points

Most strokes are caused by blocked arteries

Some strokes are caused by bleeding

TIA is a temporary warning event

Symptoms can look similar in all types

Early evaluation is critical

Chapter Summary

Stroke has three main forms. Ischemic stroke occurs due to blockage of a blood vessel. Hemorrhagic stroke occurs due to bleeding in the brain. Transient ischemic attack is a temporary interruption of blood flow and serves as a warning sign.

Although these types differ in cause and treatment, their symptoms are often similar. Immediate medical evaluation is essential in all cases.

Action Plan

- Remember that all stroke symptoms require urgent action
- Never try to guess the type of stroke
- Treat a TIA as a serious warning
- Seek immediate medical care even if symptoms improve
- Share this understanding with your family

Bridge to Chapter 3

Now that you understand the different types of stroke, the next step is even more important.

Recognizing stroke in real life.

In the next chapter, we will focus on the warning signs and symptoms that you must never ignore.

CHAPTER 3: The Warning Signs: Recognize Stroke in Seconds and Act Without Delay

Why This Chapter May Save a Life

If there is one chapter I want every reader to remember, it is this one.

Stroke does not give you time to prepare. It appears suddenly, often without warning. In that moment, the person next to the patient becomes the first responder.

You do not need medical training. You need clarity and the willingness to act.

I have seen patients recover well because someone recognized the signs early. I have also seen severe disability simply because help was delayed.

The difference is often a few minutes.

Doctor's Pearl

In stroke, recognition is the first step of treatment. The sooner you recognize it, the sooner help can begin.

The FAST Rule: A Simple Tool That Works

To make recognition easy, doctors use a simple rule called FAST.

F for Face
Ask the person to smile. Does one side of the face droop or look uneven

A for Arm
Ask the person to raise both arms. Does one arm drift down or feel weak

S for Speech
Ask the person to repeat a simple sentence. Is the speech slurred or unclear

T for Time
If you notice any of these signs, call 911 immediately

Even one sign is enough to act.

Do not wait for all signs to appear.

BE FAST: A More Complete Approach

FAST is helpful, but it does not capture every stroke.

BE FAST adds two important signs.

B for Balance
Sudden loss of balance, dizziness, or trouble walking

E for Eyes
Sudden trouble seeing in one or both eyes

F for Face
Facial drooping

A for Arm
Weakness or numbness

S for Speech
Slurred or confused speech

T for Time
Call 911 immediately

This expanded approach helps detect more types of stroke.

Common Symptoms You Should Never Ignore

Stroke symptoms usually begin suddenly. This is a key clue.

Be alert for:

- Sudden weakness or numbness, especially on one side
- Sudden confusion or difficulty understanding
- Sudden trouble speaking
- Sudden vision problems
- Sudden dizziness or loss of coordination
- Sudden severe headache without clear cause

Even one of these symptoms is enough to act.

Myth vs Fact

Myth: Stroke symptoms must be severe to be important
Fact: Even mild symptoms can represent a serious stroke or warning sign

Subtle Symptoms That Are Often Missed

Not every stroke begins dramatically.

Sometimes symptoms are mild or brief.

A person may feel slight dizziness, minor speech difficulty, or temporary vision changes. These may last only minutes and then improve.

Many people ignore these signs.

This is a dangerous mistake.

These may represent a TIA or early stroke.

Ignoring them removes the chance for early treatment.

Stroke in Women: A Slightly Different Pattern

Women may sometimes present with less typical symptoms.

These may include:

- Sudden fatigue
- Confusion
- Nausea
- Generalized weakness

Because these are less specific, they may be overlooked.

Awareness is critical.

What To Do When You Suspect a Stroke

Do not hesitate.

Take immediate action.

- Call 911 right away
- Note the exact time symptoms started
- Keep the person safe and comfortable
- Do not give food or drink
- Stay calm and stay with the person
- Unlock the door for emergency responders

Every minute matters.

Common Mistakes to Avoid

Waiting to see if symptoms improve

Driving to the hospital instead of calling 911

Giving food or home remedies

Letting the person sleep

Ignoring mild or temporary symptoms

These delays can reduce treatment options.

A Real-Life Example

A 60-year-old man noticed mild weakness in his arm and slight speech difficulty. He thought it was nothing serious and decided to rest.

A few hours later, his symptoms worsened. By the time he reached the hospital, treatment options were limited.

Another patient with similar early symptoms called 911 immediately and received timely treatment.

The difference was early recognition.

Key Points

Stroke symptoms begin suddenly

FAST and BE FAST help recognize stroke

Even mild symptoms should not be ignored

Immediate action improves outcomes

Delays increase the risk of permanent damage

Chapter Summary

Recognizing stroke symptoms quickly is one of the most important steps in protecting the brain. Stroke often begins suddenly with symptoms such as weakness, speech difficulty, vision problems, dizziness, or severe headache.

Simple tools like FAST and BE FAST make recognition easy. Immediate action, especially calling 911, can significantly improve outcomes.

BE FAST: SPOT A STROKE SAVE A LIFE

Learn the signs. Act fast. Every minute counts.

B — **BALANCE**
Sudden loss of balance, dizziness or trouble walking.

E — **EYES**
Sudden trouble seeing in one or both eyes.

F — **FACE**
Ask the person to smile. Does one side of the face droop?

A — **ARMS**
Ask the person to raise both arms. Does one arm drift down?

S — **SPEECH**
Ask the person to repeat a simple sentence. Is their speech slurred or strange?

T — **TIME**
Time to call 911 immediately. Note the time symptoms started.

CALL 911 IMMEDIATELY
Quick action can save brain cells and save lives.
DON'T WAIT. ACT FAST.

Action Plan

- Memorize the FAST and BE FAST signs
- Teach these signs to your family
- Decide now that you will call 911 immediately
- Never ignore mild symptoms
- Keep emergency numbers easily accessible

Bridge to Chapter 4

Now that you know how to recognize stroke, the next step is understanding why it happens.

In the next chapter, we will explore the major risk factors and how controlling them can protect your brain and your future.

CHAPTER 4: Why Stroke Happens: Understanding the Risks You Can Change and the Ones You Cannot

Why This Chapter Matters

Stroke rarely happens without a reason.

In most patients, it is the final result of a long, silent process that develops over many years. Blood vessels gradually become damaged. Narrowing develops. Clots become more likely. In some cases, vessels weaken and may rupture.

By the time a stroke occurs, the groundwork has already been laid.

The encouraging truth is this.

Many of these risk factors can be identified early and controlled effectively. When you understand them clearly, you gain the power to prevent a stroke or reduce the risk of another one.

Doctor's Pearl

Stroke is often the visible result of invisible damage that has been building quietly over years.

The Silent Process Inside Blood Vessels

Inside your arteries, especially those supplying the brain, a gradual process takes place.

The inner lining becomes damaged. Fatty deposits begin to collect. Over time, these deposits form plaques that narrow the artery and reduce blood flow.

These plaques can become unstable. When that happens, a clot can form suddenly and block the artery.

This process is called atherosclerosis.

The important point is that you usually feel nothing during this stage.

Everything seems normal.

Then one day, a blockage or rupture occurs, and the stroke happens.

High Blood Pressure: The Most Important Risk Factor

Among all risk factors, high blood pressure is the most important.

It damages blood vessels, accelerates plaque formation, and increases the risk of both blockage and bleeding in the brain.

The challenge is that high blood pressure often causes no symptoms.

Many people feel perfectly well while damage continues.

This is why it is called a silent condition.

Controlling blood pressure is the single most effective way to reduce stroke risk.

Diabetes: Gradual Damage to Blood Vessels

Diabetes affects both large and small blood vessels.

High blood sugar damages the inner lining of arteries, increases inflammation, and accelerates atherosclerosis.

Over time, this increases the risk of clot formation.

Patients with poorly controlled diabetes have a significantly higher risk of stroke.

Good control can greatly reduce this risk.

Cholesterol: Fuel for Plaque Formation

Cholesterol plays a major role in plaque formation.

When levels are high, fatty deposits accumulate in the artery walls.

This leads to narrowing and instability.

If a plaque ruptures, a clot can form quickly and block blood flow.

Managing cholesterol helps reduce plaque buildup and stabilizes existing plaques.

MAJOR STROKE RISK FACTORS

Some factors can increase your risk of stroke.
The good news: many of them can be controlled.

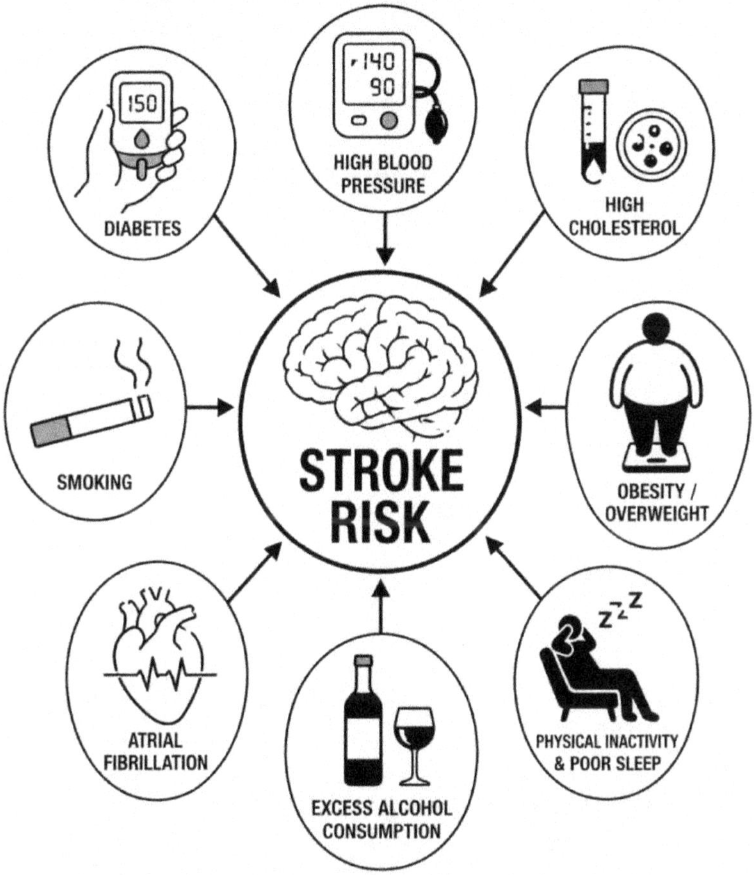

Control the risk factors.
Protect your brain. Prevent stroke.

Smoking: A Major and Preventable Cause

Smoking damages blood vessels in multiple ways.

It increases inflammation, promotes clot formation, reduces oxygen delivery, and raises blood pressure.

Even light smoking increases stroke risk.

The good news is that quitting smoking reduces risk significantly, and benefits begin early.

Obesity and Physical Inactivity

Excess body weight, especially around the abdomen, increases the risk of high blood pressure, diabetes, and abnormal cholesterol.

Physical inactivity worsens these problems.

A sedentary lifestyle slows circulation and affects overall health.

Regular physical activity improves multiple risk factors at the same time.

Atrial Fibrillation: A Heart Rhythm That Increases Risk

Not all strokes begin in the brain.

In atrial fibrillation, the heart beats irregularly. Blood can pool in the heart and form clots.

These clots can travel to the brain and cause stroke.

Strokes related to this condition are often severe, but they are highly preventable with proper treatment.

Alcohol and Substance Use

Excessive alcohol intake raises blood pressure and increases stroke risk.

Certain drugs can sharply increase blood pressure and trigger stroke.

Moderation and avoidance are important.

Non-Modifiable Risk Factors

Some risk factors cannot be changed.

These include:

Increasing age

Family history of stroke

Genetic factors

You cannot modify these, but you can be more careful about controlling the risks you can change.

The Combined Effect of Risk Factors

Most patients do not have just one risk factor.

They may have slightly elevated blood pressure, borderline diabetes, and mild cholesterol issues.

Individually, these may seem minor.

Together, they significantly increase stroke risk.

Managing all risk factors together provides stronger protection.

Myth vs Fact

Myth: If I feel fine, I am not at risk
Fact: Many risk factors, especially high blood pressure and cholesterol, cause no symptoms

A Real-Life Example

A 55-year-old man had mild blood pressure elevation and slightly high cholesterol. He felt well and did not take these seriously.

Over time, these untreated conditions damaged his blood vessels, and he suffered a stroke.

Another patient with similar findings followed medical advice, made gradual lifestyle changes, and remained stroke-free.

The difference was awareness and action.

Key Points

Stroke often results from long-term vessel damage

High blood pressure is the most important risk factor

Diabetes and cholesterol contribute to risk

Smoking significantly increases risk

Obesity and inactivity worsen multiple factors

Atrial fibrillation increases clot risk

Multiple risk factors together increase overall risk

Chapter Summary

Stroke is usually the result of long-term damage to blood vessels. High blood pressure, diabetes, high cholesterol, smoking, obesity, and inactivity are major risk factors. Atrial fibrillation and certain lifestyle factors also play important roles.

Although some risk factors cannot be changed, many can be controlled. Managing these consistently can significantly reduce stroke risk.

Action Plan

- Check your blood pressure regularly
- Monitor blood sugar if at risk
- Get cholesterol evaluated and managed
- Stop smoking completely
- Increase physical activity
- Work toward a healthy weight
- Limit alcohol intake
- Discuss heart rhythm issues with your doctor

Bridge to Chapter 5

Now that you understand why stroke happens, the next step is to understand how it affects the body.

In the next chapter, we will explore how stroke impacts movement, speech, memory, emotions, and daily life.

CHAPTER 5: How Stroke Affects the Body: Movement, Mind, and Everyday Life

Why This Chapter Matters

When we say "stroke affects the brain," it sounds limited.

In reality, the effects are widespread.

The brain is the control center of the body. It directs movement, speech, thinking, vision, balance, swallowing, and emotions. When any part of the brain is injured, the effects appear in daily life, often suddenly and dramatically.

Understanding these effects helps reduce fear, improves early recognition, and allows better planning for recovery.

Doctor's Pearl

After a stroke, the question is not only what is lost, but also what can be regained with time and effort.

Movement and Strength: When the Body Does Not Respond

Weakness on one side of the body is one of the most common effects of stroke.

This happens because the brain sends signals to muscles through specific pathways. When these pathways are damaged, the signal becomes weak or absent.

You may notice:

- Weakness in the arm, leg, or both on one side
- Difficulty standing or walking
- Poor coordination
- Reduced hand control

Some patients gradually regain strength. Others may have partial recovery.

Early rehabilitation plays a key role in improving outcomes.

Over time, some patients may develop muscle stiffness, called spasticity, which requires targeted therapy.

Speech and Language: When Communication Becomes Difficult

Stroke can affect communication in different ways.

Aphasia is a language problem. A person may know what they want to say but cannot express it properly. Others may have difficulty understanding spoken words.

Dysarthria is a speech problem caused by weak or uncoordinated muscles, leading to slurred speech.

These conditions can be frustrating.

With speech therapy and patience, many patients improve.

Swallowing: A Hidden but Serious Risk

Swallowing is a complex function controlled by the brain.

After a stroke, swallowing may become unsafe.

Food or liquids can enter the airway instead of the stomach. This is called aspiration and can lead to serious lung infection.

Because of this risk, swallowing is carefully assessed before eating.

Depending on the situation:

- Some patients eat normally
- Some need modified food
- Some require temporary feeding support

This step is essential for safety.

Doctor's Pearl

Never assume swallowing is normal after a stroke. It must be checked before eating.

Vision and Balance: Losing Orientation

Stroke can affect vision and balance.

Patients may experience:

- Loss of vision on one side
- Double vision
- Difficulty judging distance
- Dizziness or imbalance

Some patients are not aware of their vision loss.

Balance problems increase the risk of falls and require careful attention.

Thinking and Memory: Changes in Cognition

Cognitive changes are common.

These may include:

- Memory problems
- Reduced attention
- Slower thinking
- Difficulty planning or making decisions

Simple tasks may become more challenging.

With structured routines and therapy, improvement is possible.

Emotions and Behavior: The Invisible Impact

Stroke affects emotions as well as the body.

Patients may experience:

- Depression
- Anxiety
- Irritability

- Sudden mood changes

These changes may result from both emotional stress and brain injury.

Addressing emotional health is essential for recovery.

Myth vs Fact

Myth: Stroke recovery is only physical
Fact: Emotional and cognitive recovery are equally important

Daily Life and Independence

Stroke can affect basic activities such as:

- Dressing
- Bathing
- Eating
- Walking
- Managing medications
- Handling daily tasks

Loss of independence can be difficult.

However, many patients regain independence with time and rehabilitation.

Impact on Family and Caregivers

Stroke affects the entire family.

A family member often becomes a caregiver. Responsibilities increase. Daily routines change.

Caregivers may experience stress and fatigue.

Recognizing this impact early helps in planning support.

A Real-Life Example

A 65-year-old patient developed weakness and speech difficulty after a stroke.

Initially, he needed help with walking, eating, and communication.

With consistent therapy and family support, he gradually improved. He regained some independence and could communicate basic needs.

His recovery was steady, not immediate.

Key Points

Stroke affects multiple body systems

Weakness and coordination problems are common

Speech and language difficulties may occur

Swallowing problems can lead to complications

Vision and balance issues increase fall risk

Cognitive and emotional changes are important

Stroke affects both the patient and the family

HOW STROKE AFFECTS THE BODY

A stroke can affect different parts of the brain.
This can change the way you think, move, speak and feel.

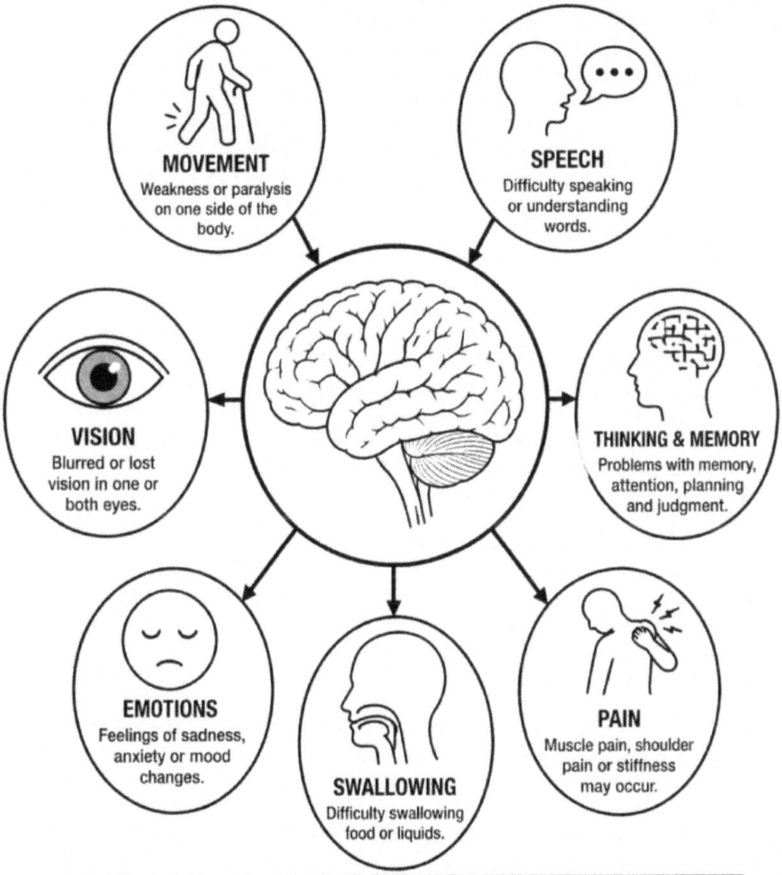

Every stroke is different.

Early treatment and rehabilitation can improve recovery.

Chapter Summary

Stroke affects not only the brain but also movement, communication, thinking, emotions, and daily life. The effects vary depending on the location and severity of brain injury.

Understanding these changes helps guide recovery and improves long-term outcomes. With rehabilitation and support, many patients regain meaningful function.

Action Plan

- Be aware of the wide range of stroke effects
- Support early rehabilitation
- Follow swallowing precautions carefully
- Encourage communication with patience
- Monitor emotional health
- Make the home environment safe
- Support caregivers

Bridge to Chapter 6

Now that you understand how stroke affects the body, the next step is to understand what happens immediately after symptoms begin.

In the next chapter, we will walk through the emergency response and why each minute matters.

CHAPTER 6: From 911 to the Emergency Room: What Happens in Those Critical Minutes

Why This Chapter Matters

In stroke care, minutes matter.

I have seen patients who acted quickly and received timely treatment. Their recovery was often remarkable. I have also seen patients who waited, hoping symptoms would improve, only to lose valuable time.

Stroke care is a race against time.

This chapter will walk you through exactly what happens from the moment you call 911 to the time you reach the hospital. When you understand this process, you will act with confidence, not hesitation.

Doctor's Pearl

The decision to call 911 is often the most important step in stroke care.

The First Step: Calling 911

If you suspect a stroke, call 911 immediately.

Do not wait. Do not try to confirm the diagnosis.

When you call:

- The dispatcher will ask simple questions
- You may be asked to check speech or movement
- Emergency services are sent right away

This call activates a rapid response system.

What Emergency Services Do

When emergency personnel arrive, they begin evaluation immediately.

They check:

- Consciousness
- Speech
- Strength and movement
- Blood pressure and pulse

They use simple stroke assessment tools.

If stroke is suspected:

- They provide basic care
- They transport the patient quickly
- They alert the hospital in advance

This early alert saves time.

Why Ambulance Transport Matters

Many people think it is faster to drive to the hospital.

In most cases, calling an ambulance is better.

This is because:

- The hospital is alerted before arrival
- The stroke team is ready
- Evaluation begins immediately

This reduces delay in treatment.

Arrival at the Emergency Room

At the hospital, everything moves quickly.

The stroke team is often already prepared.

Within minutes:

- A brief history is taken
- The time of symptom onset is confirmed
- A focused neurological exam is done

One question is very important:

"When was the patient last seen normal?"

This determines treatment options.

Imaging: The First Critical Test

A brain scan is done immediately, usually a CT scan.

This helps answer a key question:

Is the stroke caused by blockage or bleeding?

This distinction is essential for treatment.

In many hospitals, this scan is completed within minutes.

Rapid Decision-Making

Once the type of stroke is identified, treatment decisions are made quickly.

If it is a blocked artery:

- Clot-dissolving medicine may be given

If there is a large blockage:

- A procedure to remove the clot may be considered

If it is bleeding:

- Treatment focuses on controlling the bleeding

These decisions are time-sensitive.

Common Mistakes That Cause Delay

Certain actions can delay treatment.

These include:

- Waiting at home
- Ignoring symptoms
- Not noting the time of onset
- Driving instead of calling 911

Avoiding these mistakes preserves treatment options.

WHAT TO DO IN A STROKE EMERGENCY

Act FAST. Every minute can save brain cells and save lives.

1 **RECOGNIZE THE SIGNS**

Look for BE FAST signs:
Balance, Eyes, Face, Arms,
Speech, Time.

2 **CALL 911 IMMEDIATELY**

Do not wait. Call emergency services right away.

3 **NOTE THE TIME**

Note the exact time when symptoms started.
This is very important.

4 **KEEP THE PERSON SAFE AND COMFORTABLE**

Do not give food or drink.
Keep them calm and reassure them.

5 **GO TO THE HOSPITAL**

The person will receive the right treatment as quickly as possible.

QUICK ACTION. RIGHT ACTION.
BETTER OUTCOME.
DON'T DELAY. CALL 911.

WHAT NOT TO DO DURING A STROKE

1. DO NOT GIVE FOOD OR DRINK
2. DO NOT GIVE ANY MEDICINE
3. DO NOT MOVE THE PERSON UNLESS NECESSARY
4. DO NOT DELAY GETTING HELP
5. DO NOT LEAVE THE PERSON ALONE
6. DO NOT WASTE TIME WAITING TO SEE IF SYMPTOMS IMPROVE

ACT FAST. SAVE LIVES.

A Real-Life Example

A 62-year-old woman developed slurred speech and weakness.

Her family called 911 immediately.

She reached the hospital quickly and received timely treatment, leading to good recovery.

Another patient delayed seeking help and lost the chance for early treatment.

The difference was time.

Key Points

Calling 911 activates rapid care

Emergency teams begin evaluation immediately

Hospitals prepare before the patient arrives

Imaging determines the type of stroke

Treatment decisions depend on timing

Delays reduce treatment options

Chapter Summary

The first minutes after a stroke are critical. Calling 911 immediately allows rapid evaluation and early treatment. Emergency teams and hospitals work together to reduce delays and improve outcomes.

Early action significantly increases the chance of recovery.

Action Plan

- Call 911 immediately if stroke is suspected
- Do not wait or delay
- Note the time symptoms started
- Use emergency services instead of driving
- Stay calm and support the patient

Bridge to Chapter 7

Once the patient reaches the hospital, the next step is to confirm the diagnosis and identify the cause.

In the next chapter, we will explore the tests used to diagnose stroke and how they guide treatment and prevention.

CHAPTER 7: Diagnosing Stroke and Finding the Cause: Getting the Full Picture

Why This Chapter Matters

When a patient reaches the hospital with suspected stroke, speed is essential.

But speed alone is not enough.

Accuracy matters just as much.

Doctors must answer three critical questions, often within a very short time:

Is this truly a stroke
What type of stroke is it
What caused it

These answers guide immediate treatment and long-term prevention.

In my experience, many patients improve after the initial event but do not complete the full evaluation. That is a missed opportunity.

Treating the stroke is only the first step. Understanding the cause is what prevents the next one.

Doctor's Pearl

A stroke is not fully treated until its cause is clearly identified and addressed.

The First Step: Brain Imaging

The most urgent test in stroke evaluation is brain imaging.

In most hospitals, the first test is a CT scan of the brain.

This scan is fast and widely available. Its main purpose is to detect bleeding.

The key question is simple:

Is there bleeding in the brain or not

If bleeding is present, certain treatments must be avoided. If there is no bleeding, doctors can move forward with treatments to restore blood flow.

In some cases, an MRI may also be performed.

MRI provides more detailed information and can detect smaller or earlier changes in brain tissue.

Doctor's Pearl

The first brain scan guides the entire direction of treatment.

Looking at the Blood Vessels

Doctors often evaluate the blood vessels supplying the brain.

This helps identify where the problem is and how severe it is.

Common tests include:

- CT angiography
- MR angiography
- Carotid ultrasound

These tests can show:

- Narrowed arteries
- Blocked vessels
- Reduced blood flow

This information helps guide further treatment.

Blood Tests: Understanding the Body

Blood tests are done early.

They help:

- Check blood sugar
- Assess kidney function
- Evaluate clotting ability
- Measure cholesterol

They also help rule out conditions that can mimic stroke.

For example, low blood sugar can produce stroke-like symptoms.

Heart Evaluation: Searching for the Source

In some patients, stroke begins in the heart.

An ECG checks the heart rhythm and helps detect atrial fibrillation.

Sometimes, irregular rhythms are not constant, so longer monitoring may be needed.

An echocardiogram, which is an ultrasound of the heart, may also be performed.

This helps detect:

- Clots in the heart
- Valve problems
- Structural abnormalities

Finding a heart-related cause is important because it changes long-term treatment.

Carotid Artery Evaluation

The carotid arteries in the neck supply blood to the brain.

These arteries can become narrowed due to plaque buildup.

Evaluation may include:

- Carotid ultrasound
- CT angiography
- MR angiography

Significant narrowing increases stroke risk and may require specific treatment.

Looking for Less Common Causes

In some patients, especially younger individuals, the cause may not be obvious.

Doctors may look for:

- Blood clotting disorders
- Inflammatory conditions
- Rare vascular problems

A thorough evaluation ensures nothing important is missed.

Why Finding the Cause Matters

Different causes require different treatments.

For example:

- Stroke from atrial fibrillation requires anticoagulants
- Stroke from artery narrowing may need a procedure
- Stroke from uncontrolled blood pressure requires strict control

Without identifying the cause, prevention becomes incomplete.

Common Mistake to Avoid

Feeling better and skipping further testing.

Recovery does not mean the risk is gone.

A Real-Life Example

A 70-year-old patient presented with stroke symptoms.

Initial imaging confirmed the diagnosis. Further testing revealed atrial fibrillation.

He was started on appropriate treatment, reducing his risk of another stroke.

Without this evaluation, his future risk would have remained high.

Key Points

Stroke diagnosis involves confirmation and cause identification

CT scan is usually the first test

MRI provides more detailed information

Blood vessel imaging identifies narrowing or blockage

Heart evaluation is essential in many patients

Finding the cause is critical for prevention

Chapter Summary

Diagnosing stroke involves confirming its presence and identifying its cause. Brain imaging, especially CT scan, plays a central role in early decision-making. Additional tests evaluate blood vessels, heart function, and other possible causes.

This comprehensive approach allows doctors to select the correct treatment and prevent future strokes.

Action Plan

- Understand that stroke evaluation involves multiple tests
- Provide accurate information about symptom onset
- Complete all recommended tests
- Ask your doctor about the cause of your stroke
- Follow up regularly

Bridge to Chapter 8

Now that you understand how stroke is diagnosed and its cause identified, the next step is treatment.

In the next chapter, we will discuss emergency treatments that can restore blood flow or control bleeding and improve outcomes when given in time.

CHAPTER 8: Emergency Treatment: Saving the Brain When Every Minute Counts

Why This Chapter Matters

Once a stroke is recognized and diagnosed, everything becomes urgent.

This is the moment when treatment can change the course of a person's life.

I have seen patients walk out of the hospital with minimal weakness because treatment was given in time. I have also seen patients left with significant disability because that window was missed.

Emergency treatment is not about doing everything. It is about doing the right thing, at the right time, for the right patient.

Doctor's Pearl

In stroke care, the clock starts when symptoms begin, not when the patient reaches the hospital.

The Goal of Emergency Treatment

The goal is clear.

Save as much brain tissue as possible.

In a blocked artery, this means restoring blood flow quickly.
In bleeding, it means controlling the bleeding and protecting the brain.

Every decision in the emergency room is guided by this principle.

Clot-Dissolving Treatment: Opening the Blocked Artery

In ischemic stroke, where a clot blocks a blood vessel, doctors may use clot-dissolving medication.

This treatment works by breaking down the clot and restoring blood flow.

When given early and in the right patient, it can significantly improve recovery.

However, it is not suitable for everyone.

Doctors consider:

- Time since symptoms began
- Type of stroke
- Overall condition
- Risk of bleeding

Doctor's Pearl

Clot-dissolving treatment can be life-changing, but timing is critical.

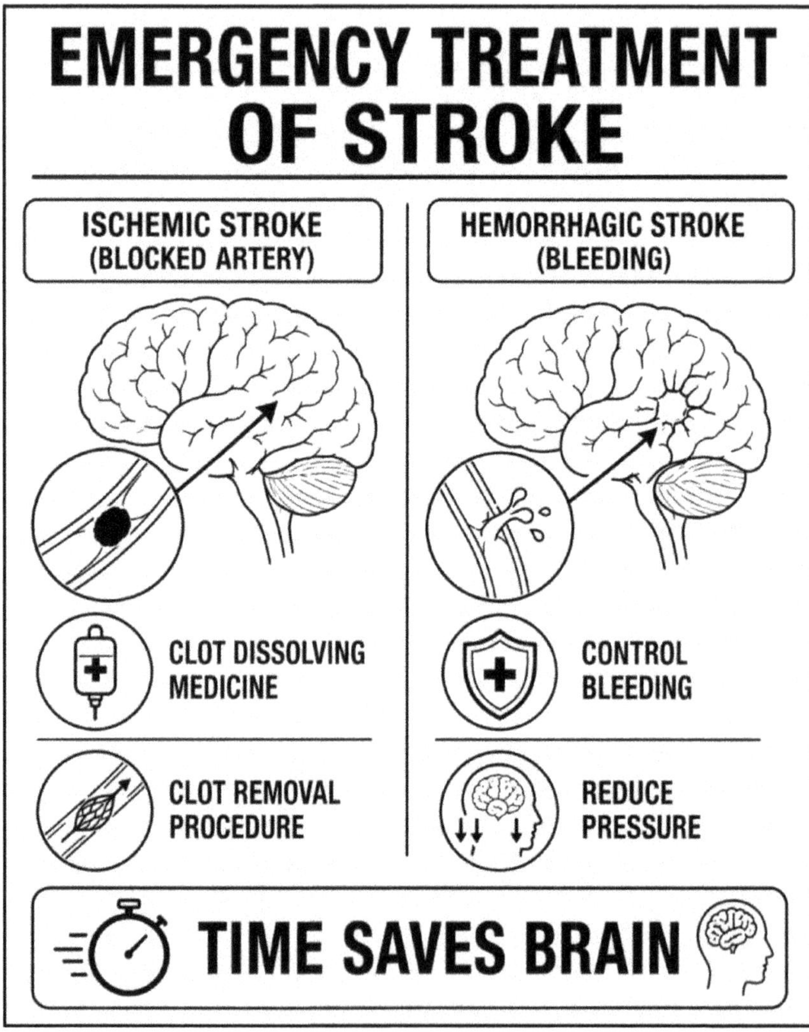
EMERGENCY TREATMENT OF STROKE
ISCHEMIC STROKE
(BLOCKED ARTERY)
HEMORRHAGIC STROKE
(BLEEDING)
CLOT DISSOLVING MEDICINE
CONTROL BLEEDING
CLOT REMOVAL PROCEDURE
REDUCE PRESSURE
TIME SAVES BRAIN

Mechanical Thrombectomy: Removing the Clot

For some patients, especially those with large artery blockages, a procedure called mechanical thrombectomy is performed.

In this procedure:

- A thin tube is inserted through an artery, usually from the groin or wrist
- It is guided to the blocked artery in the brain
- A device is used to remove the clot

This has transformed stroke care.

In selected patients, it can restore blood flow even several hours after symptoms begin.

Myth vs Fact

Myth: If treatment is delayed, nothing can be done
Fact: Some patients may still benefit from advanced procedures depending on timing and imaging

Treatment of Hemorrhagic Stroke

When stroke is caused by bleeding, the approach is different.

The focus is on:

- Controlling the bleeding
- Reducing pressure in the brain
- Preventing further damage

Doctors may:

- Carefully control blood pressure
- Reverse blood-thinning medications
- Monitor closely

In some cases, surgery is required.

Each case is unique.

Blood Pressure Management During Stroke

Blood pressure is managed carefully during stroke.

In some ischemic strokes, slightly higher pressure may be allowed temporarily to maintain blood flow.

In hemorrhagic stroke, blood pressure is usually lowered more aggressively.

This balance is managed by the medical team.

Understanding Risks and Benefits

Every treatment has risks and benefits.

Clot-dissolving medication can restore blood flow but carries a risk of bleeding.

Procedures can remove clots but involve procedural risks.

Doctors use established guidelines to make safe and effective decisions.

Common Mistakes That Reduce Treatment Options

Delays can limit treatment.

Common mistakes include:

- Waiting at home
- Ignoring early symptoms
- Not knowing the time of onset
- Delaying medical care

Avoiding these mistakes preserves treatment options.

A Real-Life Example

A 58-year-old patient developed sudden weakness and difficulty speaking.

His family acted quickly and called 911.

He reached the hospital in time, received treatment, and recovered with minimal disability.

Another patient delayed and lost the opportunity for early treatment.

The difference was timing.

Key Points

Emergency treatment aims to save brain tissue

Clot-dissolving medicines restore blood flow

Mechanical thrombectomy removes large clots

Bleeding strokes require control of bleeding

Blood pressure is carefully managed

Early action improves outcomes

Chapter Summary

Emergency treatment focuses on protecting the brain by restoring blood flow in blocked strokes or controlling bleeding in hemorrhagic strokes. Treatments such as clot-dissolving medication and thrombectomy have improved outcomes significantly.

Timing is the most important factor.

Action Plan

- Recognize stroke as an emergency
- Call 911 immediately
- Do not delay
- Note the time symptoms begin
- Understand that early treatment improves recovery

Bridge to Chapter 9

After emergency treatment, the focus shifts to stabilization and early recovery.

In the next chapter, we will explore what happens in the first few days in the hospital and how this phase influences long-term outcomes.

CHAPTER 9: The First Days After Stroke: Stabilization, Safety, and the Start of Recovery

Why This Phase Matters

After the emergency treatment is completed, there is often a sense of relief.

The patient has reached the hospital. Immediate care has been given.

But the journey is far from over.

The first few days after a stroke are critical. During this time, the brain is still vulnerable. Complications can develop. At the same time, the earliest stages of recovery begin.

What happens in these days often shapes the long-term outcome.

Doctor's Pearl

The first few days after a stroke are not just about survival. They are about setting the direction of recovery.

Where Care Happens: Stroke Units and Intensive Care

Most patients are admitted to a stroke unit or, in more serious cases, an intensive care unit.

Stroke units are specially designed for stroke care.

They provide:

- Continuous monitoring
- Coordinated team care
- Early rehabilitation support

The care team may include doctors, nurses, physical therapists, speech therapists, and other specialists.

Patients treated in stroke units often have better outcomes.

Close Monitoring: Watching for Changes

During the first few days, the patient's condition can change.

The medical team closely monitors:

- Level of consciousness
- Strength and movement
- Speech and understanding
- Blood pressure and heart rhythm
- Oxygen levels

Even small changes can be important.

Early detection allows early treatment.

Preventing Complications: A Key Goal

Preventing complications is a major focus.

Common complications include:

Lung infection due to swallowing problems

Blood clots in the legs due to reduced movement

Bed sores from immobility

Urinary infections

Brain swelling

To reduce these risks, the care team focuses on:

- Early movement
- Proper positioning
- Skin care
- Blood clot prevention
- Breathing support when needed

Preventing complications improves recovery.

Swallowing and Nutrition: A Critical Step

Swallowing is evaluated early.

If swallowing is unsafe, food or liquids can enter the airway and cause infection.

Based on the assessment:

- Some patients eat normally
- Some need modified diets
- Some require temporary feeding support

This ensures safety and proper nutrition.

Doctor's Pearl

Always assess swallowing before allowing food or drink after a stroke.

Early Movement: Starting Rehabilitation

In the past, patients were kept in bed longer.

We now know that early movement helps recovery.

As soon as it is safe, patients are encouraged to:

- Sit up
- Stand with support
- Begin simple exercises

Early movement:

- Improves circulation
- Prevents complications
- Stimulates brain recovery

Even small steps matter.

Emotional Reactions: The Human Side

Stroke can be emotionally overwhelming.

Patients may feel:

- Confused
- Anxious

- Frustrated
- Fearful

Families may also feel stressed.

Clear communication and reassurance are important.

Emotional support helps recovery.

The Role of Family

Families play an important role from the beginning.

They can:

- Provide emotional support
- Help communicate patient needs
- Understand the care plan
- Prepare for the next phase

Involvement improves outcomes.

Planning the Next Step

Planning for the next stage begins early.

This may include:

- Transfer to a rehabilitation center
- Discharge home with therapy
- Additional support services

The goal is a smooth transition.

A Real-Life Example

A 68-year-old patient was admitted after a stroke with weakness and swallowing difficulty.

Early assessment led to a modified diet. Movement began within a few days.

Because complications were prevented and rehabilitation started early, recovery progressed steadily.

Key Points

The first few days are critical

Stroke units provide specialized care

Close monitoring detects complications early

Preventing complications improves outcomes

Swallowing must be assessed early

Early rehabilitation supports recovery

Chapter Summary

The early hospital phase focuses on stabilization, preventing complications, and beginning recovery. Stroke units provide organized care that improves outcomes.

Early monitoring and early rehabilitation are key to better recovery.

Action Plan

- Understand that recovery begins in the hospital

- Stay informed about the patient's condition
- Support early rehabilitation
- Follow advice on diet and movement
- Monitor emotional health
- Prepare for the next stage

Bridge to Chapter 10

While early care focuses on stabilization, complications can still develop.

In the next chapter, we will discuss these complications and how to prevent or manage them effectively.

CHAPTER 10: Complications After Stroke: What Can Go Wrong and How to Stay One Step Ahead

Why This Chapter Matters

After the initial emergency, many patients and families feel that the danger has passed.

In reality, this phase still requires careful attention.

Stroke is not just a single event. It is a process that continues over days and weeks. During this time, several complications can develop. Some are mild. Others can delay recovery or become serious.

The encouraging part is this.

Most complications can be prevented or managed when they are recognized early.

Doctor's Pearl

Good stroke care is not only about treating the event. It is about preventing what comes next.

Brain Swelling: Pressure Inside the Skull

After a significant stroke, the brain tissue may swell.

Since the skull cannot expand, pressure builds up. This can affect healthy parts of the brain.

Warning signs include:

- Increasing drowsiness
- Worsening weakness
- Severe headache
- Vomiting

The medical team monitors closely for these signs.

Treatment may include medications to reduce swelling. In some cases, surgery is required.

Aspiration Pneumonia: A Preventable Risk

Swallowing problems are common after stroke.

If food or liquids enter the airway, it can lead to lung infection.

Warning signs include:

- Coughing during meals
- Fever
- Breathing difficulty

Prevention includes:

- Swallowing assessment before eating
- Modified diet if needed
- Eating in an upright position
- Supervision during meals

With proper care, this complication can often be avoided.

Deep Vein Thrombosis: Clots in the Legs

Reduced movement slows blood flow in the legs.

This can lead to clot formation.

These clots can travel to the lungs and become dangerous.

Prevention includes:

- Early movement
- Leg exercises
- Compression devices
- Blood-thinning medications when appropriate

Simple measures make a big difference.

Falls: A Common but Preventable Risk

Weakness, balance problems, and vision changes increase fall risk.

Falls can cause injury and delay recovery.

Prevention includes:

- Assisted walking
- Use of walking aids
- Removing obstacles at home
- Good lighting

Preventing falls is essential.

Depression and Emotional Changes

Emotional health is often overlooked.

Patients may experience:

- Depression
- Anxiety
- Loss of motivation
- Irritability

These changes affect recovery.

Early recognition and treatment improve outcomes.

Myth vs Fact

Myth: Feeling low after stroke is normal and does not need treatment
Fact: Depression is common but treatable, and addressing it improves recovery

Recurrent Stroke: The Most Important Risk

After one stroke, the risk of another increases.

This risk is highest in the first weeks and months.

Prevention becomes a priority.

This includes:

- Taking medications regularly
- Controlling blood pressure
- Managing diabetes and cholesterol

- Following lifestyle changes

Consistency is essential.

Long-Term Disability

Some patients may have lasting effects such as:

- Weakness
- Speech problems
- Memory issues
- Reduced independence

Recovery varies.

With rehabilitation, many patients improve significantly.

Common Mistakes to Avoid

Ignoring swallowing precautions

Avoiding movement due to fear

Skipping medications

Ignoring emotional symptoms

Underestimating mild problems

Awareness helps prevent these mistakes.

A Real-Life Example

A patient recovering from stroke developed coughing during meals.

Initially ignored, it progressed to pneumonia and delayed recovery.

Another patient followed swallowing precautions and avoided this complication.

The difference was early attention.

Key Points

Complications can affect recovery

Brain swelling requires monitoring

Swallowing problems can lead to pneumonia

Reduced movement increases clot risk

Falls are preventable

Emotional health matters

Risk of another stroke is high

Chapter Summary

Complications after stroke can influence recovery and long-term outcome. These include brain swelling, lung infection, blood clots, falls, emotional changes, and recurrent stroke.

Most complications can be prevented or managed with early recognition and proper care.

Action Plan

- Be aware of possible complications
- Follow medical advice carefully
- Ensure safe swallowing practices
- Encourage safe movement
- Prevent falls
- Monitor emotional health
- Focus on preventing another stroke

Bridge to Chapter 11

Preventing complications is essential, but recovery is equally important.

In the next chapter, we will focus on rehabilitation and how patients regain strength, function, and independence.

CHAPTER 11: Rehabilitation: Rebuilding the Brain and Regaining Independence

Why This Chapter Matters

After the emergency phase and early stabilization, a new and very important phase begins.

Recovery.

This is the stage where patients and families often ask:

"How much can I recover?"

The honest answer is this.

Recovery depends on several factors, but one of the most important is rehabilitation.

Rehabilitation is not an optional step. It is the central pathway through which recovery happens.

I have seen patients regain independence with steady effort. I have also seen lost opportunities when rehabilitation was delayed or inconsistent.

Doctor's Pearl

The brain has a remarkable ability to adapt. Rehabilitation helps guide that recovery.

Neuroplasticity: The Brain's Ability to Relearn

The brain is not fixed.

It has the ability to reorganize and form new connections. This is called neuroplasticity.

After a stroke, healthy areas of the brain can sometimes take over lost functions.

New pathways can develop. Existing ones can strengthen.

This ability is strongest in the early weeks and months.

That is why early rehabilitation is so important.

Starting Early: The Right Approach

Rehabilitation usually begins as soon as the patient is medically stable, often within one to two days.

Early therapy helps:

- Prevent muscle stiffness
- Improve circulation
- Reduce complications
- Stimulate brain recovery

Even small movements in the beginning are meaningful.

Common Mistake to Avoid

Waiting until the patient feels stronger before starting therapy.

Early, guided activity is part of recovery.

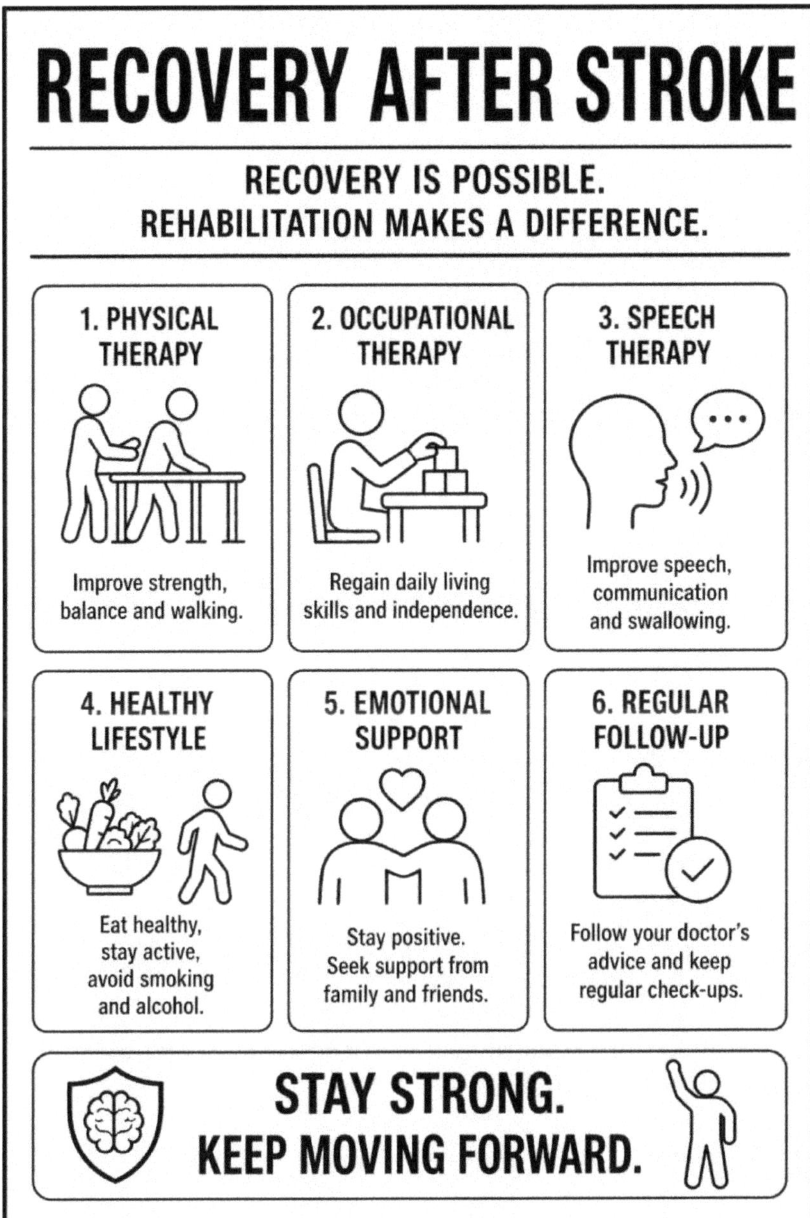
RECOVERY AFTER STROKE
RECOVERY IS POSSIBLE.
REHABILITATION MAKES A DIFFERENCE.
1. PHYSICAL THERAPY
Improve strength, balance and walking.
2. OCCUPATIONAL THERAPY
Regain daily living skills and independence.
3. SPEECH THERAPY
Improve speech, communication and swallowing.
4. HEALTHY LIFESTYLE
Eat healthy, stay active, avoid smoking and alcohol.
5. EMOTIONAL SUPPORT
Stay positive. Seek support from family and friends.
6. REGULAR FOLLOW-UP
Follow your doctor's advice and keep regular check-ups.
STAY STRONG.
KEEP MOVING FORWARD.

Physical Therapy: Restoring Movement

Physical therapy focuses on movement and strength.

The goals include:

- Improving muscle strength
- Enhancing balance
- Increasing coordination
- Helping the patient walk safely

Progress may feel slow, but even small improvements matter.

Consistency is essential.

Occupational Therapy: Regaining Daily Skills

Occupational therapy focuses on daily activities.

These include:

- Dressing
- Bathing
- Eating
- Using hands effectively
- Managing simple daily tasks

Therapists help patients relearn these skills or find new ways to perform them.

Small adaptations can make a big difference.

Speech and Language Therapy: Rebuilding Communication

Stroke can affect communication.

Speech therapy helps patients:

- Improve speech clarity
- Understand language
- Communicate effectively
- Address swallowing problems

Improvement takes time, but steady practice leads to progress.

Family support is very important.

Cognitive Rehabilitation: Improving Thinking and Memory

Stroke can affect memory, attention, and decision-making.

Cognitive rehabilitation focuses on:

- Improving memory
- Increasing attention
- Enhancing problem-solving

Simple strategies such as routines and repetition help.

Mental recovery is as important as physical recovery.

Emotional Recovery: Healing the Invisible Wounds

Stroke affects emotions as much as it affects the body.

Patients may experience:

- Depression
- Anxiety
- Frustration
- Loss of confidence

These feelings are very real.

Sometimes they come from the stress of the event. Sometimes they are directly related to changes in the brain.

Emotional health is not a secondary issue.

It directly affects motivation, participation in therapy, and overall recovery.

Support, counseling, and sometimes medication may be needed.

Myth vs Fact

Myth: Recovery stops after a few months
Fact: Improvement can continue for a long time with ongoing effort and support

Setting Realistic Expectations

Recovery after stroke is different for every person.

Some patients improve quickly. Others take longer. Some may have lasting limitations.

A common pattern is:

- Faster improvement in the early weeks
- Gradual progress over months
- Slower gains over time

It is important to remain patient and celebrate small improvements.

Recovery is a journey, not a single event.

The Role of Family and Caregivers

Family support is one of the strongest factors in recovery.

Caregivers can:

- Encourage regular therapy
- Assist with exercises
- Provide emotional support
- Help maintain daily routines

At the same time, caregivers need rest and support.

Balanced care helps both the patient and the caregiver.

Where Rehabilitation Takes Place

Rehabilitation can occur in different settings:

- Inpatient rehabilitation centers
- Skilled nursing facilities
- Outpatient therapy programs
- Home-based therapy

The goal is to provide the right level of care based on the patient's needs.

A Real-Life Example

A 63-year-old patient developed weakness and speech difficulty after a stroke.

Initially, he needed help with basic activities.

With regular therapy and family support, he gradually improved. He regained strength, improved communication, and became more independent.

His progress was steady, not immediate.

Key Points

Rehabilitation is essential for recovery

The brain can adapt through neuroplasticity

Early therapy improves outcomes

Physical, occupational, and speech therapy are key

Cognitive and emotional recovery are important

Consistency and patience are essential

Chapter Summary

Rehabilitation is the core of stroke recovery. It helps the brain relearn functions and allows patients to regain independence. Early and consistent therapy leads to better outcomes.

Recovery varies for each individual, but steady effort, emotional support, and realistic expectations can lead to meaningful improvement.

Action Plan

- Start rehabilitation as early as advised
- Participate actively in therapy
- Practice exercises regularly
- Set small, achievable goals
- Address emotional health
- Support caregivers and maintain a positive environment

Bridge to Chapter 12

Recovery is one part of the journey. Prevention is the next.

In the next chapter, we will focus on how to prevent another stroke and protect your future.

CHAPTER 12: Preventing the Next Stroke: Protecting Your Future with Clarity and Consistency

Why This Chapter Matters

After a stroke or a TIA, one question stays in every patient's mind:

"Will this happen again?"

The honest answer is yes, the risk is real.

The risk of another stroke is highest in the first few weeks and months, but it does not disappear over time unless active steps are taken.

The encouraging truth is this.

A large number of repeat strokes can be prevented.

Prevention is not complicated. But it requires clarity, commitment, and consistency.

Doctor's Pearl

The first stroke is a warning. What you do next determines your future.

Understanding the Cause: The Starting Point

The most important step in prevention is understanding why the stroke occurred.

Different causes require different strategies.

For example:

- A clot from the heart requires specific blood-thinning treatment
- Narrowed arteries may require a procedure
- High blood pressure requires strict control

Make it a habit to ask your doctor:

"What caused my stroke, and what should I do to prevent another one?"

Blood Pressure Control: The Most Powerful Step

If I had to choose one factor, it would be blood pressure.

High blood pressure damages blood vessels and increases the risk of both blockage and bleeding.

Many patients feel normal even when their blood pressure is high.

Regular monitoring and proper treatment are essential.

Consistent control significantly reduces stroke risk.

Diabetes Management: Protecting Blood Vessels

Diabetes damages blood vessels over time.

High blood sugar increases inflammation and accelerates atherosclerosis.

Effective management includes:

- Regular monitoring
- Medication adherence
- Healthy diet
- Regular follow-up

Good control reduces risk.

Cholesterol Control: Stabilizing Arteries

High cholesterol leads to plaque buildup in arteries.

Managing cholesterol helps:

- Reduce new plaque formation
- Stabilize existing plaques
- Lower the risk of clot formation

Treatment may include diet, exercise, and medications.

Smoking: A Risk That Must Be Eliminated

Smoking is a major risk factor.

It damages blood vessels, increases clot formation, and raises blood pressure.

Stopping smoking is one of the most effective preventive steps.

Benefits begin early.

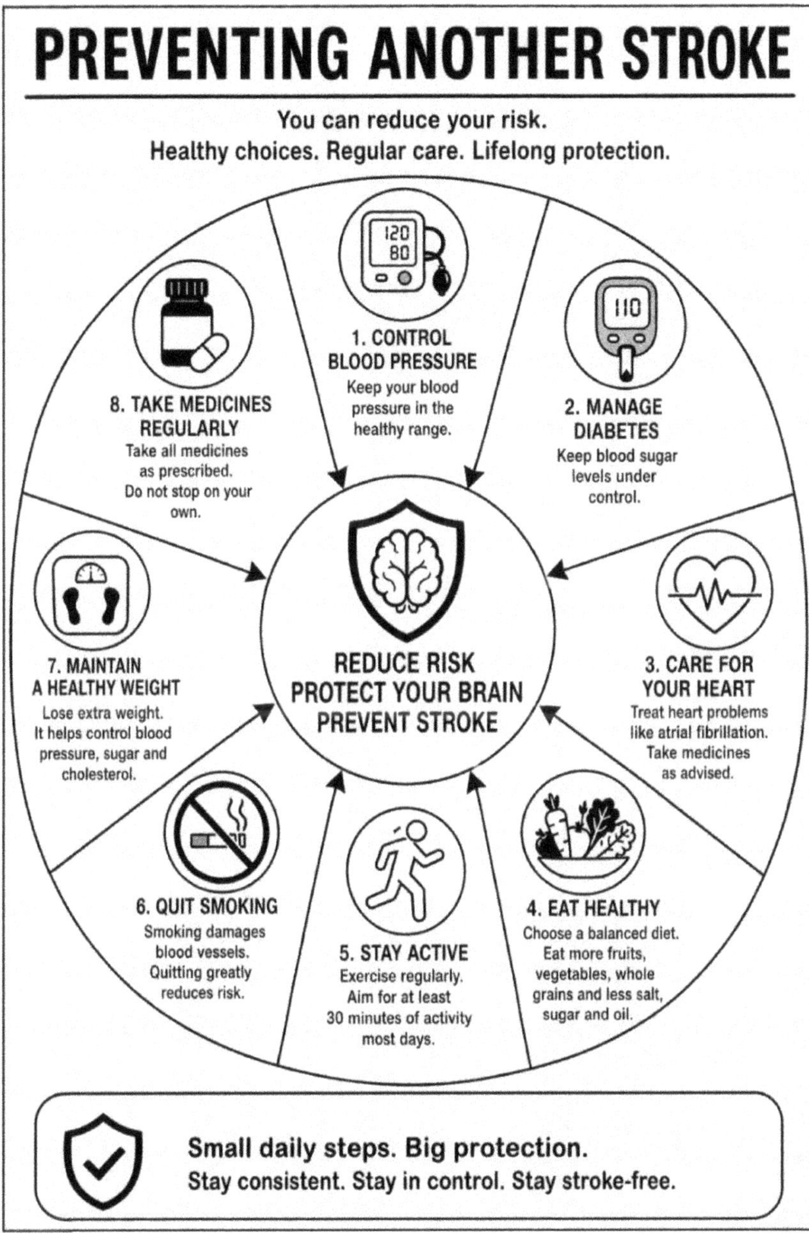
PREVENTING ANOTHER STROKE
You can reduce your risk.
Healthy choices. Regular care. Lifelong protection.
120
80
1. CONTROL BLOOD PRESSURE
Keep your blood pressure in the healthy range.
110
2. MANAGE DIABETES
Keep blood sugar levels under control.
3. CARE FOR YOUR HEART
Treat heart problems like atrial fibrillation. Take medicines as advised.
4. EAT HEALTHY
Choose a balanced diet. Eat more fruits, vegetables, whole grains and less salt, sugar and oil.
5. STAY ACTIVE
Exercise regularly. Aim for at least 30 minutes of activity most days.
6. QUIT SMOKING
Smoking damages blood vessels. Quitting greatly reduces risk.
7. MAINTAIN A HEALTHY WEIGHT
Lose extra weight. It helps control blood pressure, sugar and cholesterol.
8. TAKE MEDICINES REGULARLY
Take all medicines as prescribed. Do not stop on your own.
REDUCE RISK
PROTECT YOUR BRAIN
PREVENT STROKE
Small daily steps. Big protection.
Stay consistent. Stay in control. Stay stroke-free.

Physical Activity: A Daily Protective Tool

Regular activity improves multiple risk factors.

It helps:

- Lower blood pressure
- Improve blood sugar
- Improve cholesterol
- Maintain healthy weight

Simple activities like daily walking are very effective.

Consistency matters more than intensity.

Healthy Diet: A Practical Approach

A balanced diet supports long-term health.

Focus on:

- Fruits and vegetables
- Whole grains
- Lean proteins
- Reduced salt
- Limited processed foods

Small, consistent improvements are more effective than extreme diets.

Weight Management: Steady Progress

Excess weight increases stroke risk.

Even modest weight loss improves blood pressure, diabetes, and cholesterol.

Aim for gradual, sustainable progress.

Atrial Fibrillation and Heart Health

If stroke is related to atrial fibrillation, specific treatment is needed.

This often includes anticoagulant medication.

Regular follow-up is essential.

Medication Adherence: The Foundation of Prevention

Medications are essential.

They are not optional.

These may include:

- Blood thinners
- Blood pressure medicines
- Cholesterol medications
- Diabetes medications

Skipping medicines increases risk.

Myth vs Fact

Myth: I feel better, so I can stop my medicines
Fact: Feeling better often means treatment is working

Regular Medical Follow-Up

Prevention requires ongoing care.

Regular follow-up allows:

- Adjustment of medications
- Monitoring of risk factors
- Early detection of problems

Stay connected with your doctor.

A Real-Life Example

A 62-year-old patient had a mild stroke.

He followed medical advice, took medicines regularly, improved diet, and started daily walking.

He remained stroke-free.

Another patient did not follow through and suffered another stroke.

The difference was consistency.

Key Points

Risk of another stroke is significant

Understanding the cause is essential

Blood pressure control is most important

Managing diabetes and cholesterol reduces risk

Smoking cessation is critical

Lifestyle changes are powerful

Medications must be taken regularly

Follow-up care is essential

Chapter Summary

Preventing another stroke is a central goal after the first event. This involves understanding the cause and managing key risk factors such as blood pressure, diabetes, cholesterol, and lifestyle habits.

Medications and consistent healthy habits provide strong protection.

Action Plan

- Ask about the cause of your stroke
- Monitor blood pressure regularly
- Manage diabetes and cholesterol
- Stop smoking
- Begin regular physical activity
- Improve diet step by step
- Take medications as prescribed
- Attend regular follow-up visits

Bridge to Chapter 13

Prevention involves both lifestyle and medical treatment.

In the next chapter, we will focus on medications, how they work, and why they are essential for long-term protection.

CHAPTER 13: Medicines That Protect the Brain: Clarity, Confidence, and Consistency

Why This Chapter Matters

After a stroke, many patients go home with several medicines.

This often leads to a natural question:

"Do I really need all of these?"

It is a fair question.

In my experience, patients follow treatment much better when they clearly understand the purpose of each medicine. When the reason is clear, the treatment becomes meaningful.

These medicines are not just for the past event. They are protecting your future.

Doctor's Pearl

The right medicine, taken regularly, is one of the strongest protections against another stroke.

Antiplatelet Medicines: Preventing Clots in Arteries

Antiplatelet medicines reduce the ability of platelets to stick together.

Platelets help stop bleeding, but when they clump inside arteries, they can form clots.

These medicines help prevent that process.

They are commonly used in patients who have had an ischemic stroke not related to a heart rhythm problem.

Their goal is simple:

Prevent new clots from forming in arteries.

They are usually taken long term.

Anticoagulants: Preventing Clots from the Heart

Anticoagulants are often called blood thinners, although they do not actually thin the blood.

They reduce the blood's ability to clot.

These medicines are especially important in atrial fibrillation.

In this condition, blood can pool in the heart and form clots, which can travel to the brain.

Anticoagulants significantly reduce this risk.

Because they are powerful, they require careful monitoring.

Myth vs Fact

Myth: Blood thinners are too dangerous
Fact: When used correctly, they greatly reduce stroke risk

Statins: More Than Cholesterol Control

Statins are known for lowering cholesterol, but they also provide additional benefits.

They help:

- Stabilize plaques
- Reduce inflammation
- Lower clot risk

Even patients with normal cholesterol may benefit after a stroke.

Blood Pressure Medicines: The Cornerstone

Controlling blood pressure is the most important step in prevention.

Many patients need medication to achieve this.

Often, more than one medicine is required.

Consistency is essential.

Missing doses can lead to fluctuations and increase risk.

Diabetes Medicines: Protecting Blood Vessels

For patients with diabetes, medications help control blood sugar.

Good control protects blood vessels and reduces stroke risk.

These may include tablets or insulin.

Regular use is important.

Why Multiple Medicines Are Needed

It is common to take more than one medicine.

Each one targets a different risk factor.

For example:

- One prevents clot formation
- One controls blood pressure
- One lowers cholesterol

Together, they provide stronger protection.

Understanding Side Effects Without Fear

All medicines can have side effects.

Common ones may include:

- Mild stomach discomfort
- Easy bruising
- Fatigue

Serious side effects are less common.

The benefit of preventing stroke usually outweighs these risks.

Never stop medication without medical advice.

Common Mistake to Avoid

Stopping medicines because you feel better.

Feeling better often means treatment is working.

Medication Adherence: The Real Challenge

One of the biggest challenges is not prescribing medicines. It is taking them regularly.

Patients may skip doses because:

- They feel well
- They forget
- They worry about side effects

Irregular use reduces protection.

Practical Ways to Stay Consistent

Simple strategies help:

- Use a pill organizer
- Set reminders
- Take medicines at the same time daily
- Keep a written list
- Involve family members

Consistency is key.

MEDICINES THAT HELP PREVENT STROKE

These medicines reduce your risk of another stroke.
Take them as prescribed. Do not stop on your own.

1. BLOOD THINNERS

Help prevent blood clots.

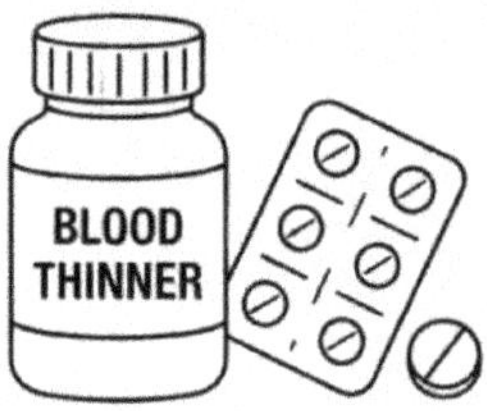

- Aspirin
- Clopidogrel
- Warfarin
- Newer Blood Thinners (e.g., Apixaban, Rivaroxaban)

2. BLOOD PRESSURE MEDICINES

Help keep blood pressure in the safe range.

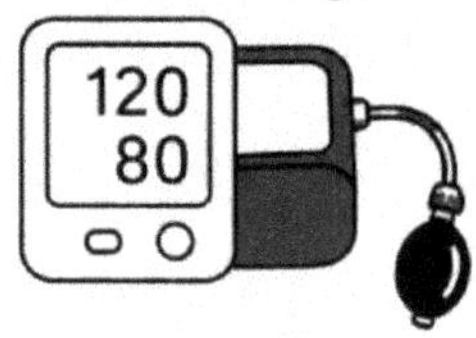

- ACE Inhibitors
- ARBs
- Calcium Channel Blockers
- Diuretics
- Beta Blockers

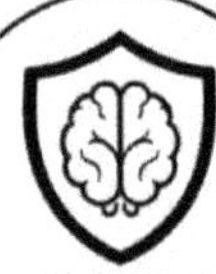

PROTECT YOUR BRAIN

3. CHOLESTEROL LOWERING MEDICINES

Help reduce bad cholesterol and protect blood vessels.

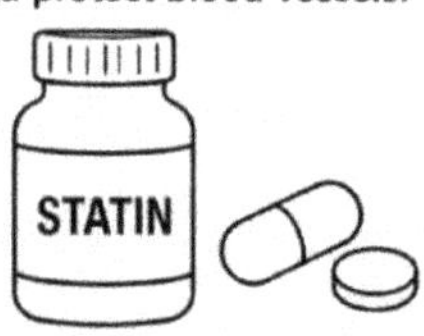

- Statins (e.g., Atorvastatin, Rosuvastatin)
- Other medicines if needed

4. DIABETES MEDICINES

Help control blood sugar and reduce stroke risk.

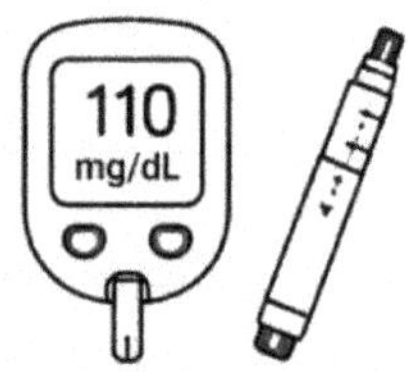

- Metformin
- Other oral medicines
- Insulin (if required)

Take medicines every day.
Follow your doctor's advice.
Regular check-ups keep you safe.

A Real-Life Example

A 68-year-old patient started skipping medicines because he felt well.

Within a year, he suffered another stroke.

Another patient remained consistent and stayed stroke-free.

The difference was adherence.

Key Points

Medicines are essential for stroke prevention

Antiplatelets prevent clots in arteries

Anticoagulants prevent clots from the heart

Statins protect blood vessels

Blood pressure medicines control the most important risk

Diabetes medicines protect vascular health

Regular use is critical

Chapter Summary

Medications play a central role in preventing stroke. Different medicines target different risk factors such as clot formation, blood pressure, cholesterol, and blood sugar.

Understanding their purpose improves adherence and protection.

Action Plan

- Understand each medicine you take
- Take medicines exactly as prescribed
- Do not stop without medical advice
- Use reminders or organizers
- Report side effects
- Stay consistent

Bridge to Chapter 14

While medicines are essential, some patients require additional treatment.

In the next chapter, we will discuss procedures and surgical options and when they are needed.

CHAPTER 14: Procedures and Surgery: When Targeted Intervention Makes the Difference

Why This Chapter Matters

For many patients, stroke prevention can be achieved with medicines and lifestyle changes.

But not always.

In some cases, there is a specific structural problem such as a severely narrowed artery or an unstable plaque that requires direct treatment.

In these situations, a carefully chosen procedure can significantly reduce the risk of a major stroke.

The key is proper selection.

Not every patient needs a procedure. But in the right patient, at the right time, it can be life-changing.

Doctor's Pearl

Procedures do not replace good medical care. They complement it when a specific problem needs direct correction.

Carotid Artery Disease: A Common Cause

The carotid arteries in the neck supply blood to the brain.

Over time, plaque can build up inside these arteries.

This can:

- Narrow the artery
- Reduce blood flow
- Create unstable areas where clots can form

These clots can travel to the brain and cause stroke.

When narrowing becomes significant, especially after symptoms, intervention may be needed.

Carotid Endarterectomy: Removing the Plaque

Carotid endarterectomy is a surgical procedure.

During this procedure:

- The artery is opened
- The plaque is removed
- Blood flow is restored

This procedure has strong evidence behind it.

In selected patients, it significantly reduces stroke risk.

Carotid Stenting: A Less Invasive Option

Carotid stenting is a minimally invasive alternative.

In this procedure:

- A catheter is inserted through an artery
- A stent is placed in the narrowed area
- The stent keeps the artery open

This may be preferred in patients who are at higher risk for surgery.

The choice depends on age, anatomy, and overall health.

Myth vs Fact

Myth: Surgery is always more risky than medical treatment
Fact: In selected patients, procedures can reduce stroke risk significantly

Procedures for Hemorrhagic Stroke

When stroke is caused by bleeding, the approach is different.

In some cases, surgery is needed to:

- Remove collected blood
- Reduce pressure in the brain
- Prevent further damage

Not all patients need surgery, but in certain situations, it can be life-saving.

Aneurysm Treatment: Preventing Bleeding

An aneurysm is a weak, bulging area in a blood vessel.

If it ruptures, it can cause severe bleeding.

If detected early, treatment may be recommended.

Two main options:

Surgical clipping
The aneurysm is closed during surgery

Endovascular coiling
Coils are placed inside the aneurysm through a catheter

Both methods aim to prevent rupture.

Weighing Risks and Benefits

Every procedure carries risk.

Possible risks include:

- Bleeding
- Infection
- Stroke during the procedure

At the same time, not treating a serious problem also carries risk.

Doctors carefully balance:

- Severity of the condition
- Expected benefit
- Patient's overall health

These decisions are made with patient and family involvement.

Common Mistake to Avoid

Delaying a recommended procedure without understanding the reason.

Ask questions and make an informed decision.

Recovery After Procedures

Recovery depends on the procedure.

Some patients recover quickly. Others need more time.

Even after a successful procedure:

- Medications are continued
- Lifestyle changes remain important
- Follow-up is necessary

A procedure corrects one problem. It does not replace long-term care.

A Real-Life Example

A 66-year-old patient had severe narrowing in a carotid artery after a minor stroke.

He underwent surgery, and blood flow improved.

With continued treatment, he remained stroke-free.

Another patient delayed treatment and later suffered a major stroke.

The difference was timely action.

Key Points

Some patients need procedures in addition to medicines

Carotid artery disease is a common reason

Endarterectomy removes plaque

Stenting is a less invasive option

Surgery may be needed in bleeding strokes

Aneurysms can be treated to prevent rupture

Decisions are based on risk and benefit

Chapter Summary

Procedures and surgery play an important role in selected patients with stroke or high risk. Conditions such as carotid artery narrowing and aneurysms may require direct treatment.

These are used along with medicines and lifestyle changes to reduce risk.

Action Plan

- Ask if you have significant artery narrowing
- Understand your treatment options
- Discuss risks and benefits
- Do not delay important decisions
- Continue medications and lifestyle changes
- Attend follow-up visits

Bridge to Chapter 15

While procedures help selected patients, long-term protection depends largely on daily habits.

In the next chapter, we will focus on lifestyle changes that truly work.

CHAPTER 15: Lifestyle Medicine: The Daily Habits That Protect Your Brain for Life

Why This Chapter Matters

If I had to choose one chapter that quietly determines long-term success, it would be this one.

Medicines help. Procedures help. Doctors guide.

But what you do every single day, often in small and simple ways, has the greatest long-term impact.

I have seen patients transform their health with steady lifestyle changes. I have also seen patients lose the benefit of good treatment because daily habits did not change.

The difference is not dramatic effort.

It is consistent effort.

Doctor's Pearl

Your daily habits are either building protection or building risk.

Eating for Brain Health: Keep It Practical

You do not need a complicated diet.

Simple, sustainable eating works best.

Focus on:

- More vegetables and fruits
- Whole grains instead of refined grains
- Lean protein such as fish, beans, and nuts
- Less salt
- Fewer processed and fried foods

Reducing salt is especially important for controlling blood pressure.

Do not aim for perfection. Aim for consistency.

Common Mistake to Avoid

Starting a strict diet that cannot be maintained.

Long-term habits matter more than short-term effort.

Physical Activity: The Most Underused Medicine

Regular movement is one of the most powerful tools for stroke prevention.

It helps:

- Lower blood pressure
- Improve blood sugar
- Improve cholesterol

- Maintain healthy weight
- Improve circulation

You do not need intense exercise.

A simple plan works:

- Brisk walking for about 30 minutes most days
- Light strength exercises
- Stretching

If recovering from stroke, follow your therapy plan.

Consistency matters.

Weight Management: Small Loss, Big Benefit

Excess weight increases stroke risk.

Even modest weight loss improves blood pressure, diabetes, and cholesterol.

The goal is gradual, sustainable progress.

Healthy eating and regular activity work together.

Sleep: The Overlooked Factor

Sleep plays an important role in health.

Poor sleep can:

- Raise blood pressure
- Affect heart rhythm
- Increase risk

Aim for:

- Regular sleep schedule
- Adequate duration
- Evaluation if you snore heavily or feel tired

Good sleep supports prevention and recovery.

Stress Management: Protecting the Mind

Chronic stress affects both mind and body.

It can lead to:

- Higher blood pressure
- Poor lifestyle choices
- Reduced motivation

You cannot remove stress completely, but you can manage it.

Helpful methods:

- Deep breathing
- Spending time with family
- Engaging in hobbies
- Maintaining routine

Even a few minutes daily can help.

Smoking: The Most Important Habit to Stop

Smoking is a major risk factor.

It damages blood vessels, increases clot formation, and raises blood pressure.

Stopping smoking is one of the most powerful steps you can take.

Benefits begin early and continue over time.

Alcohol: Keep It Moderate

Excessive alcohol increases stroke risk.

If you drink, do so in moderation.

Avoid heavy or binge drinking.

Reducing alcohol improves overall health.

Building a Sustainable Routine

The key is not intensity.

It is routine.

A simple daily structure may include:

- Balanced meals
- Regular activity
- Adequate sleep
- Time for relaxation

You do not need perfection.

You need consistency.

A Real-Life Example

A 60-year-old patient with high blood pressure made small changes.

He reduced salt, started walking daily, and improved his diet gradually.

Over time, these changes became habits.

His health improved steadily.

Another patient with similar risk factors did not make changes and later had a stroke.

The difference was consistency.

Key Points

Lifestyle changes are essential

Healthy eating supports vascular health

Regular activity improves multiple risk factors

Weight control reduces risk

Sleep and stress management are important

Smoking cessation is critical

Alcohol should be limited

Consistency is key

Chapter Summary

Lifestyle habits play a central role in stroke prevention. Healthy eating, regular physical activity, weight control, good sleep, stress management, and avoiding smoking all contribute to better health.

Small, consistent changes can significantly reduce risk over time.

Action Plan

- Start with one or two small changes
- Increase activity gradually
- Improve diet step by step
- Work toward a healthy weight
- Maintain regular sleep
- Manage stress
- Stop smoking
- Limit alcohol
- Build a routine you can maintain

Bridge to Chapter 16

While these principles apply to everyone, some groups have unique risks.

In the next chapter, we will explore special situations such as stroke in women, younger adults, and older individuals.

CHAPTER 16: Special Stroke Situations: When Risk, Symptoms, and Care Are Different

Why This Chapter Matters

Stroke does not affect everyone in the same way.

Age, gender, and underlying medical conditions can change how stroke appears, how it is diagnosed, and how it should be managed.

Recognizing these differences helps in earlier diagnosis, better prevention, and more personalized care.

Doctor's Pearl

Stroke is one condition with many faces. Recognizing these differences prevents missed opportunities for early treatment.

Stroke in Women: Unique Risks and Subtle Signs

Women have certain risk factors that men do not.

These include:

- Pregnancy-related conditions
- Hormonal therapies
- Migraine with aura in some individuals
- Higher likelihood of atrial fibrillation with age

Women may also present differently.

Instead of classic symptoms, they may have:

- Sudden fatigue
- Confusion
- Nausea
- Generalized weakness

Because these symptoms are less specific, diagnosis may be delayed.

Women also tend to live longer, which increases overall stroke risk.

Awareness is important.

Stroke in Younger Adults: Often Unexpected

Stroke is commonly thought of as a disease of older adults.

However, it can occur at any age.

In younger individuals, causes may include:

- Undiagnosed heart conditions
- Blood clotting disorders
- Artery dissection
- Smoking or substance use

Because stroke is not expected, symptoms may be ignored.

This leads to delay.

Age should never be a reason to ignore symptoms.

Stroke in Older Adults: Higher Risk, Complex Decisions

Stroke risk increases with age.

Older adults often have multiple conditions such as:

- High blood pressure
- Diabetes
- Heart disease

Recovery may be slower due to reduced physical reserve.

However, meaningful recovery is still possible.

Treatment decisions require careful balance.

Rehabilitation remains important at any age.

Silent Stroke: The Hidden Problem

Not all strokes cause obvious symptoms.

Some occur without noticeable signs and are discovered later.

These are called silent strokes.

They can lead to:

- Memory problems
- Cognitive decline
- Increased risk of future stroke

They are often related to uncontrolled risk factors.

Atrial Fibrillation: A Major Preventable Cause

Atrial fibrillation is a major cause of stroke.

In this condition, the heart rhythm is irregular. Blood can pool and form clots.

These clots can travel to the brain.

Strokes related to this condition are often severe.

The good news is that they are often preventable with proper treatment.

Stroke in Diabetes and Kidney Disease

Patients with diabetes and kidney disease have higher stroke risk.

These conditions:

- Damage blood vessels
- Increase inflammation
- Affect circulation

Careful management is essential.

This includes:

- Blood sugar control
- Blood pressure management
- Regular follow-up

Common Mistake to Avoid

Assuming stroke risk is low because you are young or feel healthy.

Stroke can occur even without obvious illness.

Myth vs Fact

Myth: Stroke happens only in old age
Fact: Stroke can occur at any age

A Real-Life Example

A 45-year-old woman experienced mild speech difficulty and dizziness.

She initially ignored the symptoms.

Later evaluation showed a small stroke related to a heart condition.

With proper treatment, her future risk was reduced.

This highlights an important lesson.

Do not ignore symptoms, even if they seem mild.

Key Points

Stroke affects different groups differently

Women may have unique risks and symptoms

Stroke can occur in younger adults

Older adults have higher risk

Silent strokes can occur without symptoms

Atrial fibrillation is a major preventable cause

Diabetes and kidney disease increase risk

Chapter Summary

Stroke is not a uniform condition. Risk factors, symptoms, and outcomes vary across different groups. Women, younger adults, and older individuals may present differently and require tailored approaches.

Certain conditions such as atrial fibrillation, diabetes, and kidney disease significantly increase risk.

Action Plan

- Understand your individual risk factors
- Do not ignore unusual symptoms
- Seek medical care promptly
- Manage chronic conditions carefully
- Stay proactive about your health

Bridge to Chapter 17

Stroke care continues to evolve.

In the next chapter, we will explore recent advances and future directions in stroke care.

CHAPTER 17: The Future of Stroke Care: Real Progress, Real Hope

Why This Chapter Matters

When I look back at how stroke was treated years ago, the difference is remarkable.

There was a time when options were limited. Diagnosis was slower. Recovery was uncertain.

Today, we are in a very different place.

Treatment is faster. Decisions are more precise. Outcomes are better.

And importantly, progress is continuing.

This chapter is not about complex research. It is about what these advances mean for real patients.

Doctor's Pearl

In stroke care, faster diagnosis and faster treatment have been the biggest drivers of better outcomes.

Better Imaging: Seeing the Problem Early

Modern imaging has changed stroke care.

Today's scans can:

- Detect stroke earlier
- Distinguish between blockage and bleeding quickly
- Identify brain tissue that can still be saved

This allows doctors to make faster and more accurate decisions.

In selected patients, treatment can now be given even beyond traditional time windows.

This means more patients can benefit.

Artificial Intelligence: Supporting Rapid Decisions

Artificial intelligence is now helping in stroke care.

It can:

- Analyze brain scans quickly
- Detect subtle changes
- Alert medical teams immediately

This reduces delay.

It is important to understand that AI supports doctors, it does not replace them.

In stroke, even small time savings matter.

Expanding Treatment Options

Stroke treatment has improved significantly.

Mechanical thrombectomy has transformed care for large artery blockages.

Ongoing research is improving:

- Devices used for clot removal
- Safety of medications
- Patient selection

These advances are expanding treatment opportunities.

Neuroprotection: Protecting Brain Cells

One area of research is neuroprotection.

The goal is to protect brain cells during a stroke.

Researchers are studying treatments that may:

- Reduce damage
- Limit inflammation
- Preserve brain tissue

Many of these are still under study but show promise.

Improving Recovery: Beyond Basic Rehabilitation

Recovery is another major focus.

New approaches aim to enhance neuroplasticity.

These include:

- Advanced rehabilitation techniques

- Brain stimulation methods
- New therapies to improve nerve connections

Stem cell research is also being explored.

These areas are still developing but offer hope.

Digital Health and Remote Monitoring

Technology is improving long-term care.

Devices can monitor:

- Heart rhythm
- Physical activity
- Blood pressure

This allows early detection of problems.

Telemedicine has also improved access to specialists, especially in remote areas.

Myth vs Fact

Myth: New treatments are always better
Fact: New treatments must be carefully tested before becoming standard care

Staying Grounded: What Matters Most

While progress is exciting, the most effective strategies remain the same:

- Early recognition
- Immediate treatment

- Control of risk factors
- Consistent medication use
- Healthy lifestyle habits

These are proven and essential.

A Real-Life Perspective

Years ago, patients with severe strokes had limited options.

Today, many of these patients can benefit from advanced treatments and recover better.

This progress gives real hope.

But one truth remains unchanged.

The sooner treatment begins, the better the outcome.

Key Points

Stroke care has improved significantly

Modern imaging allows faster diagnosis

Artificial intelligence supports decision-making

Treatment options continue to expand

Research is improving recovery

Technology supports long-term care

Proven strategies remain essential

Chapter Summary

Stroke care continues to advance with improvements in imaging, treatment, and technology. Faster diagnosis and better therapies have already improved outcomes.

Ongoing research offers hope, but current proven strategies remain the foundation of effective care.

Action Plan

- Stay informed but rely on proven treatments
- Act quickly if symptoms occur
- Follow medical advice consistently
- Use available tools to monitor health
- Focus on prevention

Bridge to Chapter 18

You have now learned about stroke from its causes to its treatment and future direction.

In the final chapter, we will bring everything together into a clear and practical plan for your life ahead.

CHAPTER 18: Bringing It All Together: Clear Answers, Common Mistakes, and Your Path Forward

Why This Final Chapter Matters

You have come a long way.

You now understand what stroke is, why it happens, how to recognize it, how it is treated, and how it can be prevented.

But knowledge alone is not enough.

In real life, what matters is clarity in the moment, confidence in decisions, and consistency in daily habits.

In my experience, most patients do not struggle because information is unavailable. They struggle because of confusion, hesitation, or common misconceptions.

This chapter brings everything together in a simple and practical way.

Frequently Asked Questions

Can stroke be completely prevented

Not every stroke can be prevented, but many can be avoided by controlling risk factors such as blood pressure, diabetes, cholesterol, smoking, and lifestyle habits.

What is the single most important step

Controlling blood pressure remains the most effective step in reducing stroke risk.

Can stroke happen without warning

Yes. Stroke often occurs suddenly. However, a TIA may act as a warning sign before a major stroke.

Is recovery always possible

Recovery varies from person to person. Early treatment and rehabilitation improve the chances of better recovery.

How long does recovery take

Recovery begins within days and may continue for months or longer. Improvement can continue with effort and therapy.

Do I need to take medicines for life

Many stroke prevention medicines are long term. They provide ongoing protection.

Is stroke only a disease of older people

No. Stroke can occur at any age, although risk increases with age.

Myth vs Fact

Myth: Stroke happens only in very old people
Fact: Stroke can occur at any age

Myth: If symptoms improve, there is no need to worry
Fact: Temporary symptoms may be a warning sign

Myth: Stroke cannot be prevented
Fact: Many strokes can be prevented

Myth: Recovery stops after a few months
Fact: Improvement can continue over time

Myth: Medicines can be stopped once you feel better
Fact: Stopping medicines increases risk

Common Mistakes to Avoid

Waiting to see if symptoms improve

Ignoring mild symptoms

Not calling 911

Skipping medications

Missing follow-up visits

Returning to unhealthy habits

These mistakes are common, but preventable.

Red Flag Warnings

Call 911 immediately if there is sudden:

Weakness or numbness on one side

Difficulty speaking or understanding

Facial drooping

Vision problems

Severe dizziness or imbalance

Severe headache without clear cause

Key Points to Remember

Stroke is a medical emergency

Time is critical

Early treatment improves outcomes

Prevention is powerful

Lifestyle and medicines both matter

Awareness saves lives

Your Personal Stroke Prevention Plan

Bring everything together into a simple plan.

- Know your numbers: blood pressure, blood sugar, cholesterol
- Take medicines regularly
- Stay physically active
- Eat a healthy diet

- Maintain a healthy weight
- Stop smoking
- Limit alcohol
- Sleep well
- Manage stress
- Stay connected with your doctor

A Final Word

Stroke can change life suddenly, but it does not have to define your future.

I have seen patients rebuild their lives with determination, support, and consistent care.

The most important step is not reading this book.

It is applying what you have learned.

Small actions, repeated every day, create powerful protection.

Chapter Summary

Stroke is a serious but often preventable condition. Understanding its warning signs, risk factors, and treatments allows better outcomes. Early action, consistent medication use, and healthy lifestyle habits are key.

Avoiding common mistakes and following a clear plan can significantly reduce risk.

Action Plan

- Remember stroke warning signs
- Call 911 immediately if symptoms occur
- Follow your prevention plan daily
- Take medications as prescribed
- Maintain healthy habits
- Attend regular follow-up visits
- Share this knowledge with your family

Final Thought

You now have the knowledge to protect your brain and your future.

Use it.

Live by it.

And help others do the same.

APPENDIX 1: Your 30-Day Stroke Prevention Plan: Turning Knowledge into Daily Action

Why This Appendix Matters

You now understand stroke and how to prevent it.

But knowledge alone does not protect you.

Action does.

In my experience, many patients start with strong motivation. They try to change everything at once. Within a few weeks, the effort becomes overwhelming, and old habits slowly return.

This plan is designed differently.

It is simple, gradual, and practical.

By the end of 30 days, these habits can become part of your daily life.

Doctor's Pearl

Do not aim for perfection. Aim for consistency. Small daily steps create lasting protection.

Week 1: Awareness and a Gentle Start

Focus on understanding your current health and beginning small changes.

- Check your blood pressure at least three times this week
- If you have diabetes, monitor blood sugar regularly
- Write down all your current medications
- Start walking for 10 to 15 minutes daily
- Reduce extra salt in your meals
- Drink more water and reduce sugary drinks
- Learn and review stroke warning signs

Goal: Build awareness and start simple habits

Week 2: Building a Routine

Focus on creating structure.

- Increase walking to about 20 to 25 minutes daily
- Add at least one serving of fruits or vegetables each day
- Reduce fried and processed foods
- Set a fixed sleep and wake time
- Begin reducing portion size if overweight
- If you smoke, begin a quit plan
- Continue monitoring blood pressure and blood sugar

Goal: Create consistency

Week 3: Strengthening Control

Focus on improving control of key risk factors.

- Walk about 30 minutes most days
- Add light strength or balance exercises
- Strictly reduce salt intake
- Take medications regularly without missing doses

- Schedule or attend a doctor visit
- Limit alcohol intake
- Practice simple stress management such as deep breathing

Goal: Improve control and discipline

Week 4: Making It a Lifestyle

Focus on long-term habits.

- Maintain regular physical activity
- Follow a balanced diet consistently
- Keep a regular sleep schedule
- Continue medications regularly
- Monitor blood pressure consistently
- Review your progress
- Involve your family

Goal: Make habits part of daily life

Daily Checklist

Use a simple checklist each day.

- Took all medications
- Completed physical activity
- Ate healthy meals
- Avoided smoking
- Limited alcohol
- Slept adequately
- Managed stress

If you complete most of these most days, you are on the right track.

Common Mistake to Avoid

Trying to change everything on the first day.

Start small. Build gradually.

A Real-Life Example

A 58-year-old patient with high blood pressure started with small changes.

He began walking daily, reduced salt intake, and monitored his blood pressure.

Over time, these small steps became habits. His health improved steadily.

He did not make dramatic changes. He made consistent changes.

Key Points

Small actions lead to long-term protection

Consistency matters more than perfection

Tracking improves awareness

Gradual change is sustainable

Family support improves success

Appendix Summary

This 30-day plan helps turn knowledge into action. By focusing on small, consistent steps, you can build habits that reduce stroke risk.

The goal is not just 30 days, but a lifetime of healthier living.

Action Plan

- Start this plan today
- Track your progress
- Focus on consistency
- Involve your family
- Continue these habits beyond 30 days

Bridge to Appendix 2

You now have a practical plan to improve your health.

In the next appendix, we will focus on what to do in an emergency so you can act quickly and confidently if a stroke occurs.

APPENDIX 2: Stroke Emergency Checklist and BE FAST Guide: Act Quickly, Act Correctly

Why This Appendix Matters

In a stroke emergency, confusion is common and precious time is often lost.

I have seen families hesitate. Someone suggests waiting. Someone else feels the symptoms may pass. A few minutes quietly turn into an hour.

Those lost minutes can mean permanent brain injury.

This guide is designed to remove hesitation.

You should be able to recognize a stroke and act immediately, without doubt.

Keep this information where it is easy to see. Share it with your family.

Doctor's Pearl

In stroke, delay is dangerous. Immediate action saves brain function.

The BE FAST Guide: Recognize Stroke in Seconds

This simple tool helps you identify stroke quickly.

B for Balance
Sudden loss of balance, dizziness, or difficulty walking

E for Eyes
Sudden trouble seeing in one or both eyes

F for Face
Ask the person to smile. Does one side droop

A for Arm
Ask the person to raise both arms. Does one arm drift down

S for Speech
Ask the person to repeat a simple sentence. Is the speech slurred or unclear

T for Time
If you notice any of these signs, call 911 immediately

Even one sign is enough to act.

Emergency Action Checklist

If you suspect a stroke, follow these steps immediately.

- Call 911 without delay
- Note the exact time symptoms started
- Keep the person safe and comfortable
- Do not give food or drink
- Stay with the person and keep them calm
- Unlock the door for emergency responders
- Keep a list of medications ready if possible

Common Mistakes to Avoid

Waiting to see if symptoms improve

Driving the patient instead of calling emergency services

Giving food, water, or home remedies

Letting the person sleep

Ignoring mild or temporary symptoms

Avoiding these mistakes can save valuable time.

Preparing in Advance

Preparation makes a difference.

- Keep emergency numbers easily accessible
- Maintain a list of medications and medical conditions
- Ensure family members know stroke warning signs
- Identify the nearest hospital

Simple preparation reduces panic.

Creating a Family Plan

Every household should have a simple plan.

Decide:

- Who will call 911
- Who will stay with the patient
- Who will gather medical information

Clear roles prevent confusion.

A Real-Life Example

A man suddenly developed difficulty speaking at home.

His wife recognized the symptoms using the BE FAST guide and called 911 immediately.

He reached the hospital quickly, received timely treatment, and recovered well.

Another patient delayed seeking help and suffered a more severe outcome.

The difference was early action.

Key Points

Stroke symptoms must be recognized quickly

BE FAST is simple and effective

Immediate action improves outcomes

Delays worsen damage

Preparation improves response

Appendix Summary

This checklist provides a clear and practical way to recognize and respond to stroke. The BE FAST method helps identify symptoms quickly, and the emergency steps ensure rapid action.

Being prepared can save time and improve outcomes.

Action Plan

- Memorize the BE FAST signs
- Share this checklist with your family
- Keep emergency numbers accessible
- Be ready to act immediately
- Never delay

Bridge to Appendix 3

You now know how to respond in an emergency.

In the next appendix, we will focus on daily monitoring and how tracking your health can help you stay in control and reduce your risk over time.

APPENDIX 3: Your Daily Health Tracker: Staying Aware, Staying in Control

Why This Appendix Matters

Stroke prevention is not a one-time decision.

It is a daily commitment.

In my experience, many patients begin with strong motivation after a stroke. They take medicines regularly, follow advice, and make changes. Over time, small lapses begin. A missed dose here, a skipped walk there.

Slowly, risk begins to rise again.

Tracking is a simple but powerful tool that prevents this drift.

When you track your health, you stay aware. When you stay aware, you stay in control.

Doctor's Pearl

What you measure regularly, you manage effectively.

What to Track: Keep It Simple

You do not need to track everything.

Focus on key areas:

- Blood pressure
- Blood sugar if you have diabetes
- Medications
- Physical activity
- Weight
- Lifestyle habits

Keeping it simple makes it sustainable.

Blood Pressure Tracker: Your Most Important Number

Blood pressure is the most important number in stroke prevention.

Track it regularly.

Use a simple format:

Date
Morning reading
Evening reading
Notes

Measure at the same time each day if possible.

Bring this record to your doctor visits.

Common Mistake to Avoid

Checking blood pressure occasionally and assuming it is controlled.

Consistency matters more than isolated readings.

Medication Tracker: Daily Protection

Missing medications increases risk.

Use a simple checklist:

Date
Morning medicines taken Yes or No
Evening medicines taken Yes or No
Any side effects

A pill organizer can help.

Blood Sugar Monitoring

If you have diabetes, monitor regularly.

Track:

- Fasting levels
- Post-meal levels if advised

Look for trends, not just single numbers.

Lifestyle Tracking: Reinforcing Good Habits

Track daily habits:

Physical activity
Did you exercise

Diet
Did you follow a healthy pattern

Smoking
Did you avoid smoking

Alcohol
Did you limit intake

Sleep
Did you get adequate rest

Simple yes or no entries are enough.

Weekly Weight Check

Check weight once a week.

Do not focus on daily changes.

Look for trends over time.

Reviewing Your Progress

Tracking is useful only if reviewed.

At the end of each week:

- Review blood pressure trends
- Check medication consistency
- Assess lifestyle habits

Adjust where needed.

Share with your doctor.

Keeping It Practical

Use:

- A notebook
- A printed sheet
- A simple phone app

The best system is the one you use consistently.

A Real-Life Example

A patient tracked his blood pressure daily.

He noticed higher readings in the evening.

His doctor adjusted medications, and control improved.

Without tracking, this pattern would have been missed.

Key Points

Tracking improves awareness

Blood pressure monitoring is essential

Medication tracking prevents missed doses

Lifestyle tracking reinforces habits

Weekly review improves control

Appendix Summary

Tracking your health is a simple and effective way to stay consistent. Monitoring blood pressure, medications, and lifestyle habits keeps you proactive.

Regular review improves care and reduces risk.

Action Plan

- Start tracking blood pressure regularly
- Use a medication checklist
- Monitor blood sugar if needed
- Track lifestyle habits
- Review progress weekly
- Share records with your doctor

Bridge to Appendix 4

You now have tools to monitor your health daily.

In the final appendix, we will focus on caregivers and home safety, helping families support recovery confidently.

APPENDIX 4: Caregiver Guide and Home Safety: Supporting Recovery with Strength and Compassion

Why This Appendix Matters

Stroke recovery is rarely a solo journey.

Behind most patients, there is someone quietly carrying a great responsibility. A spouse, a child, a relative, or a close friend who becomes the caregiver.

I have seen caregivers manage medicines, assist with movement, support therapy, coordinate appointments, and provide emotional strength every single day.

Caregivers are the backbone of recovery.

At the same time, caregiving can be physically and emotionally demanding. Without proper guidance, it can lead to stress and burnout.

This appendix is designed to help caregivers provide effective care while also protecting their own well-being.

Doctor's Pearl

A supported caregiver provides better care and sustains recovery over time.

Understanding Your Role

As a caregiver, you are part of the recovery team.

Your role may include:

- Assisting with daily activities
- Supporting medication routines
- Encouraging rehabilitation exercises
- Monitoring for new symptoms
- Providing emotional reassurance

Recovery takes time. Some days will be better than others.

Patience and consistency are essential.

Safe Mobility and Fall Prevention

After a stroke, weakness and balance problems increase the risk of falls.

You can reduce this risk by:

- Assisting during walking
- Encouraging slow and steady movement
- Using walking aids if recommended

Make the home safer:

- Remove loose rugs
- Keep pathways clear
- Ensure good lighting
- Install handrails where needed

Preventing falls is critical.

Medication Management

Managing medications can be challenging.

You can help by:

- Using a pill organizer
- Setting reminders
- Ensuring medicines are taken on time
- Watching for side effects

Consistency in medication use helps prevent another stroke.

Supporting Rehabilitation at Home

Recovery continues at home.

You can:

- Encourage daily exercises
- Help practice therapy techniques
- Support communication efforts
- Celebrate small improvements

These daily efforts build progress.

Communication and Emotional Support

Stroke may affect speech and understanding.

Support communication by:

- Speaking slowly and clearly
- Allowing time for responses

- Encouraging expression

Patients may feel frustrated or anxious.

Your patience and reassurance are very important.

Common Mistake to Avoid

Focusing only on physical recovery and ignoring emotional health.

Both are equally important.

Recognizing Warning Signs

Watch for:

- New weakness
- Speech changes
- Sudden confusion
- Signs of infection
- Stroke warning signs

If you suspect a stroke, call 911 immediately.

Do not wait.

Self-Care for the Caregiver

Caregivers often neglect their own health.

This can lead to exhaustion.

Take care of yourself:

- Take regular breaks
- Maintain your own health care
- Ask for help
- Stay connected with others

Caring for yourself allows you to care for the patient.

Building a Support System

You do not have to do everything alone.

Support can include:

- Family members
- Friends
- Home health services
- Support groups

Sharing responsibility reduces stress.

A Real-Life Example

A patient recovering from stroke needed help with daily activities.

His spouse organized medications, supported exercises, and made safety changes at home.

At the same time, she took breaks and involved other family members.

This balanced approach helped both patient and caregiver.

Key Points

Caregivers are essential in recovery

Safe mobility prevents falls

Medication management requires consistency

Home rehabilitation supports progress

Emotional support improves recovery

Caregivers must take care of themselves

Support systems are important

Appendix Summary

Caregivers play a central role in stroke recovery. Their support helps patients regain strength, confidence, and independence.

At the same time, caregivers must protect their own health and seek support when needed.

Action Plan

- Understand your caregiving role
- Make the home environment safe
- Support medications and therapy
- Provide emotional encouragement
- Watch for warning signs
- Take care of your own health
- Build a support system

Final Note

Recovery after stroke is a shared journey. With patience, consistency, and support, meaningful improvement is always possible.

You now have a complete, practical guide to understanding, managing, and preventing stroke. Use it. Share it. Live by it.

Thank You and Please Review the Book

Thank you for taking the time to read this book. I sincerely hope it has helped you understand your health a little more clearly and has given you practical, everyday steps you can follow with confidence. If you found this book helpful, **I would truly appreciate it if you could leave a brief and honest review.** Even a few lines sharing your experience can make a meaningful difference. Your feedback helps other readers find reliable, trustworthy health information and supports them in making better decisions for themselves and their families.

Warm regards,

Dr Prabhat Das

Continue your Healthcare Journey with these Books

Good health is a journey, not a single step. It is not achieved in one day or with one book. That is why I created the "Better Health with Dr Das Series", with each book addressing a different common condition. If you would like easy, practical guidance on other everyday health concerns, you may wish to explore the rest of books in this series.

Books in this series:

- Better Health starts Here: A Doctor's Guide to Staying Healthy After 40
- A Doctor's Easy Guide to Understanding & Managing OBESITY
- Doctor, What DIET Is Best for Me?
- Doctor, Why Can't I Lose Weight? A Doctor's Guide to Safe & Sustainable Weight Loss)
- A Doctor's Easy Guide to GLP-1 for Obesity
- A Doctor's Easy Guide to Understanding & Managing HIGH BLOOD PRESSURE
- A Doctor's Guide to Living Well With DIABETES
- A Doctor's Guide to Understanding & Managing THYROID DISEASES
- A Doctor's Guide to Understanding & Managing HIGH CHOLESTEROL
- A Doctor's Practical Guide to HEART HEALTH After 40: How to Protect Your Heart & Live Longer
- A Doctor's Guide to Healing & Reversing FATTY LIVER DISEASE: Simple, Natural & Science-Based Steps to Reduce Liver Fat and Prevent Complications

- Control Your ACID REFLUX, HEARTBURN & GERD: A Doctor's Practical Guide that Works
- Live Comfortably with IRRITABLE BOWEL SYNDROME: A Doctor's Practical Guide to Understanding & Managing IBS
- A Doctor's Practical Guide to Understanding & Managing GALLBLADDER STONES & OTHER PROBLEMS
- Take Control of COPD: A Doctor's Practical Guide to Better Breathing
- Living Better with ASTHMA: A Doctor's Practical Guide to Asthma Control
- SLEEP APNEA, INSOMNIA & OTHER SLEEP DISORDERS: A Doctor's Practical Guide to Better Sleep & Better Health
- Protect Your KIDNEYS: A Doctor's Practical Guide to Kidney Health & Prevention
- PROSTATE HEALTH: A Doctor's Practical Guide to Early Detection & Care
- ARTHRITIS: A Doctor's Practical Guide to Pain Control & Mobility
- STROKE: A Doctor's Practical Guide to Prevention & Early detection
- HEART ATTACK: A Doctor's Practical Guide to Prevention & Early detection
- A Doctor's Practical Guide to Fixing BACK PAIN Step by Step
- COMMON SKIN & HAIR PROBLEMS: A Doctor's Practical Guide to Skin & Hair Care
- DEMENTIA & MEMORY LOSS: A Doctor's Practical Guide to Prevention & Management
- Doctor, Why Am I TIRED All the Time? Fixing Fatigue & Getting Your Energy Back

www.ingramcontent.com/pod-product-compliance
Ingram Content Group UK Ltd.
Pitfield, Milton Keynes, MK11 3LW, UK
UKHW021959270726
14060UKWH00003B/593

9 781971 672618